Canine Clinic

Canine Clinic

THE COMPLETE GUIDE TO THE DIAGNOSIS AND TREATMENT OF YOUR DOG'S HEALTH PROBLEMS

Anna P. Clarke, D.V.M.

Illustrations by Linda McClure and Leo Gilbride

MACMILLAN PUBLISHING COMPANY   New York

Copyright © 1984 by Anna P. Clarke, D.V.M.

Illustrations by Linda McClure and Leo Gilbride

Macmillan Publishing Company
866 Third Avenue, New York, N.Y. 10022
Collier Macmillan Canada, Inc.

Library of Congress Cataloging in Publication Data

Clarke, Anna P.
Canine clinic.

Includes index.
1. Dogs—Diseases. I. Title.
SF991.C58   1984   636.7'089   84-792
ISBN 0-02-525860-5

10 9 8 7 6 5 4 3 2 1

Designed by Jack Meserole

Printed in the United States of America

I would like to dedicate this book to my late husband, Seán, who always encouraged me to write.

Reading maketh a full man, conference a
ready man, and writing an exact man.

—FRANCIS BACON, 1561–1626

Contents

Introduction

The aim of this book is to give the dog-owning public in-depth information on canine veterinary medical care and to emphasize the professionalism of the veterinarian today. Although there are many books on dog care, some by veterinarians, few really inform dog owners about canine medical problems in depth and fewer still tell them exactly what it is that veterinarians can do for their sick dogs. I hope my book will fill this gap for dog owners who want to be informed on all aspects of their dogs' medical care. Other books, after describing canine medical diseases and disorders, do not take the readers past the point of advising them to see their veterinarian. This book is presented in exactly the same way as a veterinary medical textbook written for the veterinarian; only the medical terminology has been simplified for the lay reader. Each disease is defined, followed by a discussion in detail of the cause(s), symptoms, diagnosis, treatments, prognosis, and prevention. Some people may think I go into too much technical detail, and I know some veterinarians and MDs disapprove of telling all to the client or patient, but I have found over the years, both in clinical practice and in writing about veterinary medicine, that people appreciate being well informed about their pet's or their own health care and quickly grasp the most technical information if it is presented to them clearly.

If you have read this book and take your sick dog to your veterinarian, you will probably already have some idea of what the problem is and you most certainly will be able to present an accurate medical history, which will help your veterinarian reach a diagnosis. You will understand how your veterinarian reaches a diagnosis, which tests are necessary, and what treatments are best. And most important, you will know if your dog is receiving the standard of medical care you want.

This book is not designed to help you keep your dog healthy—although early treatment and prevention of illness will certainly go a long way toward achieving this—nor is it designed to reduce your veterinary bills—but it will do so by helping you to recognize and have illnesses treated early in their course. Its purpose is to ensure that the dog owner is fully informed on a dog's medical problem and can therefore get the best medical care available for the dog.

—ANNA P. CLARKE, D.V.M.

February, 1984

1
Nutrition

WHAT TO FEED A DOG: NUTRITIONAL REQUIREMENTS

Just like people, dogs need a diet that regularly includes proteins, fats, carbohydrates, vitamins, and minerals for proper nutrition. Of equal importance is the proportioning or balance of these ingredients in the diet.

On a dry basis, an adult dog requires a minimum of 22% protein, 5.5% fat, 1.6% linoleic acid, a maximum of 67% carbohydrates, and small percentages of essential vitamins and minerals. (*See* footnote 1, Nutrient Requirements of Dogs chart, later in this chapter.)

Protein

Protein is made up of twenty-three different amino acids. The dog's body can manufacture thirteen of these, but the other ten must come from meat and plant sources. These are called "essential amino acids." Protein is used for body building; good sources are meat, eggs, milk, cheese, and plant proteins. Meat should not make up more than 25% of the dry matter of the diet. With the exception of pork and wild game, all meat can be fed raw unless the dog dislikes it that way. Eggs sould be cooked and one per each pound of food is adequate. Milk supplies calcium and phosphorus in the proper ratios, and if kept to about two fluid ounces per pound of food, it seldom causes gastrointestinal problems. Cheese is an expensive food for dogs but can be a small part of the diet.

1

Fish is an excellent protein source for dogs, but it should be cooked.

Fats and Carbohydrates

Other foods in a dog's diet are energy sources, and these are composed of fats and carbohydrates. Most fat comes from meat, but vegetable oils, such as corn oil, should also be used because they supply all the essential fatty acids. Pig, poultry, and horse fat also supply these; beef fat is quite low. Cereal grains supply the carbohydrates in a dog's diet and are used to dilute the protein. Other useful carbohydrates are potatoes, noodles, spaghetti, and macaroni. Cooking starches increases their digestion and utilization by the dog.

Vegetables and Fruits

Vegetables and fruits are not needed in a dog's diet and most vegetables are poorly digested by dogs. Some vegetables can be used if cooked.

Vitamins and Minerals

In a homemade dog diet, a good, balanced vitamin and mineral supplement is probably a wise precaution, as is the addition of one-half ounce of bone meal for every pound of meat in the diet.

ALL-MEAT DIET

Meat alone is not a good diet for a dog. In fact, a dog forced to eat nothing but meat will die. One reason so many dog owners think a meat-only diet is correct for dogs is the classification of these animals in the zoological order *Carnivora*.

This has led to the popular but erroneous assumption that dogs must therefore be strictly carnivorous (flesh-eating) animals.

Carnivora is an order, or group, of mammals that is primarily carnivorous but by no means exclusively so. This group of animals is characterized by a single stomach, a short intestine, and teeth adapted to tearing flesh. No member of this order lives exclusively on flesh, and some are even complete vegetarians. The diet of bears, raccoons, and skunks, all included in this order, is divided equally between plant and flesh foods. Only wildcats, mink, and weasels limit their food to flesh and organ meats, and even these animals consume the entire carcass of their prey. Wolves, the dog's ancestors, eat the bones and other tissues of their prey to balance their diets.

Dogs fed nothing but meat will eventually suffer from an all-meat diet syndrome known technically as nutritional secondary hyperparathyroidism. Meat not only contains very little calcium but supplies a notable imbalance of calcium and phosphorus. In meat this ratio is 1 to 20; in a normal diet for a dog this ratio should be 1.2 to 1.

If an all-meat diet is fed to a dog, the resultant abnormal levels of too little calcium and too much phosphorus in the blood stimulate the parathyroid gland to release a hormone that will correct these levels. This causes the dog's system to release calcium from the bones in order to balance the high phosphorus level. The bones are weakened by this speedy calcium withdrawal, and the result is pain, lameness, bone deformities, and even fractures. The teeth may also loosen and fall out as the bone in the jaws is depleted.

Treatment of the condition consists of correcting the diet and using a calcium supplement such as calcium carbonate. One teaspoonful of the supplement is added to the pet's diet for each pound of meat. Of course, prevention is better than treatment, so do not feed a dog an all-meat diet.

Today much of the meat protein in commercial dog foods is being replaced by plant proteins. The diminishing supply and the rising cost of meat protein are making this changeover necessary. Although these new diets are complete and balanced diets for dogs, a few dogs will not eat these new formulations, or eat them only with reluctance. This is often the case with older dogs that have eaten foods with a higher meat content all their lives.

The source of the protein for dog food does not matter very much as long as the food is balanced and nutritious for the dog. The most important factor of all, of course, is that the dog eats the food. A homemade meat-based diet (*see* later in this chapter) can be designed for a dog that will not eat commercial dog food, or complete and balanced dog food can be made more acceptable by adding meat to make the food more palatable. Do not, however, let this addition exceed 10% of the dog's daily food intake, or the nutritional balance of the commercial dog food may be upset.

VITAMIN AND MINERAL SUPPLEMENTS

There is no need to give a healthy dog vitamin and mineral supplements if it is being fed a complete and balanced dog food. These foods contain all the protein, vitamins, minerals, and other nutrients dogs are known to need, in the correct proportions. Most manufacturers of good-quality dog foods have a built-in safety margin of essential nutrients to take care of deterioration during processing and shelf storage, and also to overcome imbalances that may result when dog owners dilute these foods with table scraps or meat. These higher levels are not high enough to be toxic, but if further supplementation is added by the dog owner, problems can arise.

Supplementation Problems

More medical problems are seen in dogs today from oversupplementing with vitamins and minerals than from deficiencies. The major problem areas in over-supplementation with vitamins and minerals are: excessive vitamin D, which can lead to skeletal problems; an imbalance of the calcium and phosphorus ratio, which leads to bone abnormalities and fractures; and excessive vitamin A, which results in poor growth and painful bone disorders.

Necessary Supplements

There are exceptions, of course, and vitamin and mineral supplements are necessary:

- If signs of deficiency are evident.
- To correct a specific deficiency in dogs unable to utilize normal levels of these components in the diet.
- For hardworking dogs.
- For females during pregnancy or lactation.
- For old dogs.
- During certain illnesses where absorption is impaired, organs are damaged, or the dog is not eating.

In all these circumstances, it is best to have a veterinarian recommend the types and amounts of supplements to give the dog; it is even better to switch to a diet that will meet the dog's needs, and avoid supplements altogether.

People May Need Supplements—Dogs Generally Do Not
Although there is great interest today in the human health field in vitamin and mineral supplements, this same reasoning cannot be applied to dog nutrition because dogs eating commercial dog foods are not eating varied and imbalanced diets, as their human companions often do. Many people can justify taking supplements because their diets may be inadequate, but complete and balanced dog foods are not inadequate and therefore supplementation is more hazardous than helpful. I have emphasized this point because most dog owners do not understand this major difference between human and dog nutrition.

Vitamin Sources—Excess and Deficiency Signs

Most dog owners feeding their pets commercial dog foods do not need to concern themselves with the vitamin sources for dogs, or the signs of vitamin excesses and deficiencies. However, for those interested, the following chart outlines these sources and includes signs of deficiencies and excesses.

Vitamins for Dogs

Vitamin	Source	Deficiency Signs	Excess Signs
A	Egg yolk, liver, corn, fish oils	Poor growth, skin and bone disorders, eye problems	Weight loss, bone disorders
D	Sun, fish oils, egg yolk	Bone disorders, rickets in young	Calcium in soft tissues, loss of appetite, diarrhea
E	Egg yolk, milk, corn, cereals	Bone and muscle disorders, reproductive failure	None known. In man: lethargy and blood clotting problems
K	Liver, fish, yeast, soy beans	Blood clotting problems	None unless very high levels
C	No dietary need (synthesizes own)		None
B₁ (Thiamine)	Liver, whole grain, yeast	Poor growth, muscle weakness	None if moderate
B₂ (Riboflavin)	Milk, yeast, whole grains	Weakness, skin and eye problems, anemia	None known
Niacin	Meat, fish, eggs, whole grains	Red and ulcerated mouth, weakness, diarrhea, anemia	Dilation of blood vessels, hot and red skin

Vitamins for Dogs (*continued*)

Vitamin	Source	Deficiency Signs	Excess Signs
B$_6$ (Pyridoxine)	Meat, fish, milk, liver, whole grains	Slow growth, anemia	None known
Pantothenic Acid	Liver, rice, milk, yeast	Poor growth, diarrhea, convulsions	None known
Folic Acid	Liver, yeast	Anemia, poor appetite	None known
Biotin	No dietary need	None reported	None known
B$_{12}$ (Cocalamin)	Liver, fish, meat, milk	Anemia	None known
Choline	Liver, meat, yeast, egg yolk	Liver problems	Diarrhea

Supplements for Old Dogs

Studies have shown that proper nutrition can increase the life span of animals. There is not a great deal of scientific data available concerning nutritional supplements for the geriatric dog, but some studies have been done on the following minerals and vitamins:

Zinc. Zinc levels are decreased in the elderly, so supplementation is often used and appears helpful. Zinc promotes growth and repair at the cellular level and is needed for normal secretion and function of insulin and for normal thyroid hormone levels.

Calcium and Phosphorus. Older animals need more calcium to prevent thinning of the bones which is a problem in humans as well during old age. Also calcium is often not as readily absorbed in the intestinal tract in older animals, and excessive calcium may be lost through the urine in kidney failure. If the calcium to phosphorus ratio is upset, high phosphorus levels may lead to gum and tooth disease.

Iron. In human studies it has been found that the absorption of iron may be reduced in the elderly.

The B Vitamins. Aging is associated with lowered vitamin B levels. Signs of deficiency of one or more of the B vitamins are not unusual in older dogs. Poor appetite, loss of weight, and neurologic and cardiac problems may improve with B vitamin supplementation.

Vitamin C. Dogs synthesize their own vitamin C and are therefore seldom deficient, but it has been found that older dogs with chronic disease tend to have low levels and appear to benefit from supplementation.

Vitamin E. It has been shown in rats that their requirements for this vitamin increase with age. This has not been proven in dogs, but older dogs given this vitamin often improve in general appearance and activity.

Vitamin A. This vitamin is seldom deficient in older dogs, except for those with liver and bowel disease.

Vitamin D. High doses of vitamin D can cause severe bone problems; as dogs are seldom deficient, vitamin D is not usually recommended as a supplement except in specific deficiency cases.

In summary, vitamin and mineral supplements can often be helpful in older dogs, particularly those with chronic or debilitating diseases. Many vitamin and mineral supplements specifically designed for geriatric dogs are available. Some of these products also contain hormones that help to pep the dog up. Your veterinarian is the best source of advice on which, if any, of these products should be used.

The most important aspect of nutrition, for the old as well as the young, is a balanced diet, and there are now many special geriatric commercial dog foods available designed specifically to meet the needs of the older dog, without the addition of vitamins and minerals.

Vitamin C

As a general rule dogs do not need vitamin C in their diet. Vitamin C (ascorbic acid) has received a great deal of attention in human nutrition for a number of years, although the jury still appears to be out on whether such supplementation is beneficial or not. This vitamin is essential in the human diet to prevent the onset of scurvy. Human nutritional studies continue on the ability of vitamin C to prevent or lessen the severity of the common cold, and on its role in wound and burn healing.

Many research studies have been done on dogs in which they were deprived of dietary vitamin C, yet none of the test dogs developed scurvy. (In one study, guinea pigs which were fed the same vitamin C-deficient diet as a comparison group of puppies developed scurvy in twenty-five days, while there were no signs of scurvy in the puppies after 150 days on this diet.) In short, there is no scientific evidence that dogs require vitamin C in their diets. Dogs synthesize sufficient quantities of this vitamin to meet their bodies' needs. The synthesis takes place in the liver.

Despite these findings, some veterinary practitioners recommend vitamin C in the treatment and prevention of certain dog diseases. Although claims have been made that vitamin C is effective for treating distemper, kennel cough, cancer, hepatitis, and for preventing hip dysplasia, none of these claims have been verified in controlled scientific studies. The National Research Council has concluded that there is not adequate evidence to justify the routine addition of vitamin C to the diet of normal healthy dogs. However, in infections and certain other illnesses, the ability of the liver to manufacture ascorbic acid may become depressed, and dogs in these circumstances may need supplemental vitamin C.

TYPES OF DIETS FOR DOGS

Complete and Balanced Dog Foods

Many pet food manufacturers have put a great deal of research into the development of foods that may be safely given as a dog's sole diet without supplementation. Such foods can be identified by looking for the words "complete" or "balanced" on the label or for any statement which says the food will meet all of a dog's nutritional requirements. The use of these claims is regulated by the Federal Trade Commission, which has ruled that no manufacturer may label or advertise his product as complete or balanced unless the food "meets the National Research Council's (NRC) nutrient requirements for dogs—or—contains a combination of ingredients which, when fed to a normal dog as the only source of nourishment, will support normal growth, reproduction and adult maintenance whether working or at rest, and has had its capabilities in this regard demonstrated by adequate testing." Unfortunately, meeting the NRC requirements does not necessarily ensure that a food is adequate; it does guarantee the nutrients are present in the food in adequate amounts, but there is no guarantee they are in a form utilizable by the dog unless feeding trials are also conducted. Reputable dog food manufacturers do conduct feeding trials and will supply test results of them on request.

Of course people would find it boring to eat exactly the same one-dish meal every day even if it were a complete and balanced diet, but dogs have an entirely different attitude to food—they eat to meet their energy and body maintenance needs. At least, this is what the canine nutrition experts tell us. However, I am not too sure that dogs don't become bored with the same food every day! If one feeds a dog a wide variety of foods, it will readily adapt to this and come to expect it. The problem here is that without careful study of canine nutrition on the owner's part, the dog probably won't get a balanced and nutritious diet.

After choosing a dog food (dry, semi-moist, or canned) that is complete or balanced, it is best not to change this diet nor to add any vitamin and mineral supplements or table scraps. The trouble with table scraps is twofold: the dog may become a picky eater and he may not eat enough of his dog food to receive a complete diet. If table scraps or extra meat *are* fed, do not let this exceed 10% of the diet. Additional vitamins and minerals are not needed by the normal healthy dog on these diets and may lead to poisonous excesses or unbalanced amounts.

Two meals a day of a complete or balanced diet, with fresh water, are really all that the average dog needs to stay nutritionally healthy.

One of the most important factors in the choice of a dog food is that the food be acceptable to the dog. However, the objective should *not* be to find the most palatable food, because this can lead to obesity. The smell, taste, and texture of the food are important to a dog, but let the dog be the judge of that, as what appeals to a dog owner may not necessarily appeal to a dog. Warming canned foods and adding water to dry foods greatly enhance palatability. A recent study on taste preferences in dogs showed that they prefer beef, followed by pork, chicken, lamb, liver, and horsemeat. They prefer canned or semi-moist food to dry, canned meat to fresh, ground meat to cubed, and warmed food to cold. It seems they don't always get what they like: a study in 1981 of the type of dog food purchased disclosed that 68% was dry, 27% canned, and 5% semi-moist.

As mentioned above, dog foods that have "complete" or "balanced" or any statement on their label that they meet all of a dog's nutritional requirements must be nutritionally adequate for all the dog's needs. Because of this, it is no longer essential for dog owners to study and understand the chemical analyses on a dog food label (which are not very informative about the true value of the food), or to know much about the nutrient requirements of dogs. For those interested, the nutrient requirements for the three major types of commercial dog foods are:

Nutrient Requirements of Dogs

NUTRIENT	On a Dry[1] Basis	DOG FOODS Dry[2]	Semi-[2] Moist	Canned[2]
Water	0%	10%	25%	75%
Food Solids	100	90	75	25
Protein (minimum)	22.0%	20.0%	17.0%	6.0%
Fat (minimum)	5.5	5.0	4.0	1.4
Linoleic Acid (minimum)	1.6	1.4	1.2	0.4
Carbohydrate (maximum)	67.0	60.0	50.0	17.0
Calcium — Must be in	1.1	1.0	0.8	0.3
Phosphorus — this ratio	0.9	0.8	0.7	0.2

[1] All foods contain water. When the water is removed, measurements of the nutrient contents are made on a dry basis for scientific purposes.

[2] For ease of reference for the dog owner, the amounts of these required nutrients for the different types of dog foods are listed as they appear on a dog food label. Adjustments have been made for the varying water content of each type of dog food.

Dog Food Labeling Laws

The laws regarding the regulations affecting dog food labeling are complex and vary from state to state. The regulatory body for label disclosures on dog food sold in interstate commerce is the Federal Trade Commission (FTC), which obtains its information on nutrient requirements for dogs from the National Academy of Science of the National Research Council. Federal and state standards are also set by the Association of American Feed Control Officials (AAFCO).

The federal regulations require every dog food label to

show the following information: brand and product name, name and address of the manufacturer or distributor, the net weight, the manufacturer's guarantees for the food, the ingredients used in manufacturing the food, and whether or not the food is a nutritionally complete diet. There also should be an analysis of the product, including the minimum percentage of crude protein and fat, and the maximum percentage of crude fiber and water. Ash percentages are not required, but are usually included. Also, each ingredient used in making the food should be listed in descending order by weight.

These are general standards that apply to the pet food industry nationally. However, if a pet food is manufactured and sold only within one state, it does not come under FTC regulation. The manufacturer, however, must still comply with state pet-food laws.

Special-Purpose Dog Foods

There are three other types of commercial dog foods available:

1. *Stage-of-life dog foods.* These are commercial dog foods designed for stages of a dog's life, with diets for puppies, pregnant dogs, nursing mothers, working dogs, and old dogs. These foods meet all the nutritional requirements for the dog at the stage of life for which they are designed.

2. *Commercial dog foods which are not complete and balanced.* These are commercial dog foods which do not claim to be complete and balanced for use as the dog's sole diet, although they are nutritious foods. Most are designed as special treats for the dog or to be mixed with the dog's regular food. They should never be fed as the sole diet, nor should they make up more than 10% of the regular diet of a dog. Occasional use as a full-meal treat is acceptable.

3. *Special diets used in treating medical problems.* Like people, dogs with specific diseases often require special diets. A number of companies have designed such specialized diets, which are distributed only through veterinarians.

These foods can be slightly more expensive than regular commercial dog foods because they require special formulations and ingredients. Such diets are dispensed by veterinarians for: heart failure, kidney failure, bladder stones, digestive, pancreatic, and liver disorders, food allergy, obesity, geriatric dogs, wasting illnesses, and for heartworm, hookworm, and roundworm prevention. The following chart lists Hill's Prescription Diets, and includes their uses and nutritional characteristics:

Hill's Prescription Diets

Diet	Uses	Nutritional Characteristics
d/d	Food-induced allergies. Gastrointestinal upsets caused by diet. Test diet to diagnose a food allergy.	Protein and fat derived from sheep and rice. Carbohydrates derived from rice. Unsaturated fatty acids increased.
g/d	Older (geriatric) dog. Congestive heart failure. Hormonal imbalances.	Protein mildly restricted. Fat and carbohydrate mildly restricted. Fiber increased. Vitamins increased. Minerals mildly restricted. Unsaturated fatty acids increased. Salt mildly restricted.
h/d	Heart failure (severe). Water retention. Hypertension.	Salt severely restricted. Potassium increased. Protein mildly restricted. Fat and carbohydrate increased. Vitamins increased.
i/d	Gastrointestinal upsets. Early weaning. Pancreatic disease. Bloat.	Protein high quality. Fat restricted. Carbohydrate easily digestible. Fiber restricted. Electrolytes and vitamins increased.

Hill's Prescription Diets (*continued*)

Diet	Uses	Nutritional Characteristics
k/d	Kidney failure. Liver disease. Heart failure (mild). Hormonal imbalances. Bladder stones prevention.	Protein high quality and moderately restricted. Fat and carbohydrate increased. Minerals restricted. Vitamins increased. Sodium moderately restricted.
p/d	Nutritional deficiency diseases. Weaning and growing puppies. Gestating and lactating bitches. Diabetes mellitus (if underweight). Recuperation.	Protein increased. Fat increased. Carbohydrate decreased. Minerals increased. Vitamins increased.
r/d	Obesity. Constipation. Hypothyroidism. Diabetes mellitus (if overweight).	Fat severely restricted. Carbohydrate restricted. Fiber greatly increased.
u/d	Advanced kidney failure. Advanced liver disease. Recurrent bladder stones prevention.	Protein high quality and severely restricted. Fat and carbohydrate increased. Minerals severely restricted. Vitamins increased. Sodium moderately restricted.
s/d	Dissolves bladder stones.	Protein severely restricted. Fat and carbohydrate increased. Minerals restricted. Salt increased.
Control Diet HRH	Heartworm prevention. Eliminates roundworms and hookworms, and prevents recurrences. Working dogs.	Fat increased. Carbohydrate highly digestible. Drug additives.

Printed with permission of Hill's Pet Products, Inc.

Kidney Failure Diet

Diets for kidney failure patients are designed to decrease the demands on the kidneys. Protein, particularly meat protein, produces most of the waste material that needs to be excreted by the kidneys via the urine. The poorer the quality of the protein, the greater the amount of waste material. Dogs need some protein to live, but in kidney failure the diet must be designed to contain the minimum amount of the highest quality protein to maintain the dog in good condition.

Special canned and dry dog foods designed for dogs with kidney failure, such as Prescription Diets k/d and u/d made by Hill's are available from veterinarians, and for most dog owners this is a convenient method of controlling the diet of a dog with failing kidneys. However, a few dogs do not find these low-protein foods palatable and will not eat them. In such instances, homemade diets can be made from the following recipes:

Restricted Protein Diet	*Ultra Low-Protein Diet*
¼ pound ground beef	5 ounces or 2½ cups dry instant rice
2 cups cooked rice	1 ounce corn oil
1 hard-boiled egg	2 hard-boiled eggs
3 slices white bread	¼ teaspoon calcium carbonate
1 teaspoon calcium carbonate	Vitamin-mineral supplement to meet daily requirements
Vitamin-mineral supplement to meet daily requirements	

Braise the meat, retaining the fat to pour over the food, or in the ultra low-protein diet, cook the rice following the package directions. Combine all the ingredients and mix well. Feed as required to maintain the dog's body weight. Feed frequent small meals rather than the usual two meals a day, as this relieves the demands on the failing kidneys.

A lot of protein is lost in the urine of animals with failing kidneys, and meeting their protein requirements, without overloading the kidneys with high-protein diets, can be difficult. The meat content of the diets above may have to be adjusted by your veterinarian depending on the degree of kidney failure in the dog. As kidney failure is a slowly progressive disease, adjustments will need to be made periodically.

Dogs with kidney failure should be encouraged to drink a lot of fluids, as this maintains a high urine output, thereby flushing out waste materials.

Heart Failure Diet

Like people, dogs with heart disease require a low-sodium, low-fat diet. Special canned and dry foods, such as Prescription Diet h/d made by Hill's, are the most convenient to use. For the few dogs that will not eat these foods, a homemade diet can be made from the following recipe:

¼ pound ground round or other *lean* beef	2 teaspoons dicalcium phosphate
2 cups cooked rice	Vitamin-mineral supplement
1 tablespoon corn oil	to meet daily requirements

Cook the beef until lightly browned. Add remaining ingredients and mix well. Feed as required to maintain the dog's normal body weight. All snacks, treats, and table scraps must be eliminated.

Gastrointestinal Upset Diet

Following gastrointestinal upsets, dogs need a bland diet once the vomiting and diarrhea have been controlled. Special canned foods, such as Prescription Diet i/d made by Hill's are the most convenient to use. Alternatively, a homemade diet can be made from the following recipe:

½ cup Cream of Wheat
1½ cups creamed cottage
  cheese
1 hard-boiled egg
2 tablespoons dried brewer's
  yeast
1 tablespoon corn oil

1 tablespoon potassium
  chloride
2 teaspoons dicalcium
  phosphate
Vitamin-mineral supplement
  to meet daily requirements

Cook the Cream of Wheat following the package directions. Add remaining ingredients and mix well. Feed as required to maintain the dog's normal body weight.

Self-Feeding

Self-feeding is gaining in popularity and is used by a great many dog breeding kennels and boarding establishments. Self-feeding consists of keeping a dish or feed hopper filled with a completely balanced semi-moist or dry dog food, and allowing the dog to regulate its own intake. Semi-moist food should be put out more frequently as it tends to dry out. Fresh water, of course, must always be available.

There are a number of advantages to self-feeding dogs: it eliminates the work of preparing meals and scheduling regular feeding times; eating small amounts frequently keeps the level of nutrients more constant in the dog's bloodstream; it reduces mealtime nervousness and excitement; it reduces boredom; it often eliminates coprophagy (the habit of eating feces); in groups of dogs it allows the less aggressive dogs to get their share; and in dogs used to self-feeding, it eliminates overfilling the stomach, which may lead to a fatal stomach torsion (twisting).

There are, however, a few negative aspects to self-feeding and these include: the likelihood that some dogs will overeat and become obese, which occurs most often if they are bored or underexercised; the loss of the usually happy emotional interaction and the bonding between owners and their dogs at feeding times; the likelihood that some dogs, particularly those that have already been spoiled with specially tasty foods and table scraps, will not eat enough on self-feeding to meet their nutritional needs or will hold out for a return to special mealtime fun and favors; and the fact that foods left out for long periods of time lose some of their nutrient and vitamin values and spoil under certain hot or damp conditions.

When changing an adult dog to self-feeding, it should be done gradually over a week or more. Self-feeding is easier to establish if it is started when the dog is a puppy.

Quality of a Dog Food

Judging the quality of a commercial dog food is not an easy matter. By far the best method is to feed one food to the dog exclusively; if he thrives and looks healthy, then it is a good food. However, only complete or balanced foods should be used. Examine the dog food and if it contains a lot of grass awns, grain hulls, feathers, sand, wood chips, and other foreign material, do not buy that brand again. Small amounts of crushed bone are acceptable in dog food. The food should smell fresh. (This is particularly important for dry dog food.) If it smells rancid, do not use it; essential vitamins and fats will have been destroyed. In dog foods, as well as other things, you usually get what you pay for, and a cheap dog food may be made up of a lot of indigestible filler foods. Protein, particularly meat protein, is expensive.

A good tip on evaluating a dog food's digestibility is the amount of stool produced. If one food produces more stool than another and the stool looks like the food eaten, then it is poorly digestible and the dog owner is paying for useless food for the dog.

Homemade Diet

Our knowledge of canine nutrition is much more complete and advanced than is our knowledge of human nutrition. As a result, my fellow veterinarians and I feel we must first recommend to dog owners that they take advantage of this scientific knowledge and feed the specially formulated and guaranteed completely balanced commercial dog foods to their dogs. There is no easy formula for a homemade dog diet that can offer this same guarantee. If a dog owner is prepared to study canine nutrition, he or she can then design a variety of excellent homemade diets for the dog. A good reference source for further information on canine nutrition, available in most bookstores, is *The Collins Guide to Dog Nutrition* by Donald R. Collins, DVM, published by Howell Book House Inc., 845 Third Avenue, New York, NY 10022. This book is written for nonprofessionals, and I highly recommend it, particularly for dog owners who wish to feed their dogs a homemade diet.

A high-quality homemade maintenance diet for dogs can be made from the following recipe:

½ pound ground beef (regular, *not* lean)	3 slices white bread
	1 teaspoon calcium carbonate
1 hard-boiled egg	Vitamin-mineral supplement
2 cups cooked rice	to meet daily requirements

Cook the meat, retaining the fat. Combine all ingredients and mix well. This mixture is somewhat dry and the palatability can be improved by adding water (not milk). Feed as required to maintain the dog's normal body weight. This diet produces about 830 calories per pound.

CALORIE REQUIREMENTS OF DOGS

The calorie requirements of dogs have been determined; because of the large variations in different dog breeds' weights, one overall figure for daily calories per pound of body weight is not satisfactory. Note that small dogs need more calories per pound than large dogs.

Calorie Requirements of Dogs

Adult Dog's Weight (Pounds)	Calories Per Pound (Per Day)	Daily Calories (Total)
5	50	250
10	42	420
15	38	570
20	35	700
30	31	930
40	29	1,160
50	27	1,350
75	24	1,800
100	24	2,400
150	24	3,600

These figures are generalizations because many factors, such as age, hereditary characteristics, activity, health, climate, stress, sex, and neutering, affect calorie needs.

Calorie Content of Dog Foods

A rough approximation of the calorie content per ounce of commercial dog foods is: for dry food, 85–95; semi-moist, 80–85; canned, 31–37.

By dividing the number of calories a dog needs daily by the number of calories in an ounce of the food being fed, the number of ounces of that food needed daily can be determined. For example, a 30-pound dog needs 930 calories per day, and if fed only dry food, would need ten and one-third ounces per day (930 divided by 90).

Dog owners should feed their pets enough food to maintain them in a healthy, trim condition, rather than follow rigid daily food weight intake guidelines. If a dog owner cannot judge whether a dog is under- or overweight, then advice should be sought from a veterinarian.

OBESITY

Obesity is nearly as big a problem in dogs in the United States as it is in people. Everyone knows that 95% or more of overweight problems or obesity are caused by consuming more calories than the body requires for maintenance. It is well known that for people a reduction in physical activity is seldom associated with a reduction in food intake, and since we all tend to slow down with age, obesity is the end result for many. Some families, both human and animal, have a pre-disposition to obesity. It has been found that these subjects are highly responsive to taste and tend to overeat good-tasting foods despite being satiated. Normal individuals tend to stop eating when they are full, whether the food is tasty or not.

Other common causes of overeating in dogs today include boredom, spoiling, and lack of exercise.

Medical Effects of Obesity in Dogs

The medical problems related to obesity in dogs are the same as those seen in humans. Since nearly one-third of all dogs seen by veterinarians today are overweight, this is becoming a major factor in the practice of companion animal medicine.

Obesity is known to reduce the dog's life span. Medical problems that are related to obesity in dogs include: joint problems, such as arthritis; herniated disc and ligament rupture; respiratory difficulties, leading to fatigue and shortness of breath; congestive heart failure; decreased liver function due to fatty liver; diabetes; heat intolerance, caused by the insulating properties of excess subcutaneous fat; increased risk for surgery; lowered resistance to infectious diseases; gastrointestinal function impairment, resulting in constipation and flatulence; and increased incidence of cerebral hemorrhage (strokes).

Control of Obesity

An overweight dog should be put on a weight reduction program. There are four approaches to this: psychology, exercise, diet, and drugs. Following a physical examination of the dog to eliminate medical causes for the pet's obesity, the dog owner must then recognize that the dog is obese and must want to do something about it. It is essential to reduce the dog's calorie intake and—if there is no heart or respiratory disease present—to increase the amount of exercise. Veterinary advice is useful, although not essential if an obese dog is otherwise healthy. There are special reducing diet dog foods available from veterinarians, such as Prescription Diet r/d made by Hill's, which are designed to meet the dog's nutritional needs, while reducing the calorie intake. These special diet foods are very convenient to use. If they prefer, dog owners can reduce a dog's calorie intake by reducing the amount of food fed daily, using the dog food presently being fed (provided it is a complete and balanced dog food), until the extra pounds are shed. However, severe restriction of some dog foods may result in the dog not meeting its nutritional requirements, so it is preferable to feed the special diet foods or use a homemade diet such as the following recipe:

¼ pound of ground round or other *lean* beef
½ cup cottage cheese (uncreamed)
2 cups drained canned carrots

2 cups drained canned green beans
1½ teaspoons dicalcium phosphate
Vitamin-mineral supplement to meet daily requirements

Cook the beef until lightly browned; pour off the fat. Add the remaining ingredients and mix well. Feed daily: ⅓ pound to a 5-pound dog; ⅔ to 10 pounds; 1 to 20 pounds; 1¾ to 40 pounds; 2½ to 60 pounds; 3 to 80 pounds; and 3⅔ to 100 pounds. No snacking or scavenging should be allowed.

The use of drugs, such as appetite suppressants and thyroid hormones, is discouraged because they seldom have long-term effects, and have many undesirable side effects.

BONE CHEWING

Veterinarians are frequently asked whether or not they should allow a dog to chew bones. There is no "yes" or "no" answer; there are advantages and disadvantages to bone chewing. While dogs in the wild have to chew bones to meet their calcium and phosphorus needs, dogs receiving a complete and balanced diet do not need bones to meet their nutritional requirements. On the other hand, dogs enjoy chewing bones and this helps keep tartar from building up on their teeth. Another practical consideration is that it is better to have one's dog chew bones than furniture or shoes. When the permanent teeth begin to erupt, at about fourteen weeks of age, puppies need to chew on something to relieve their itching gums. Most dogs on reaching maturity give up this excessive chewing but will seldom turn down a juicy bone.

One disadvantage of bone chewing is that some dogs swallow a large quantity of bone, which can cause digestive upsets and even intestinal blockage. Swallowing a sharp bone splinter can cause perforation of the esophagus or intestinal tract. Another disadvantage is that excessive bone chewing can prematurely wear down, or even break a dog's teeth.

If a dog owner permits the dog to chew bones, large, hard bones such as knuckle or marrow bones should be used, of a size in proportion to the dog. If a dog manages to splinter a bone and starts swallowing parts of it, it should be taken away. Dogs should not be given bones that splinter readily, such as steak, chop, rib, or chicken bones. Rather than waste the food value of these bones, though, they can be stewed for soup for the dog. Dogs used to eating such bones very seldom get into trouble with them, but veterinarians cannot recommend their use because they see the problems these bones can cause some dogs too often.

A compromise is to allow a dog to chew on one of the many brands of cowhide bones from the pet store or supermarket. Pet stores also sell real bones, which have been cleaned and sterilized, and these can be left lying around the house without the staining problems fresh bones create.

WHY DOGS GULP FOOD

Many dog owners are distressed because their dog eats so quickly. Others often ask if such fast eating means the dog is not enjoying the food. In fact, it is normal for a dog to gulp down food hastily; this does not mean the dog is not enjoying it. It is easier to understand a dog's eating behavior if one thinks back to the ancestor of the domestic dog, the wolf. Wolves either killed game or stole game killed by other predators, and then gorged themselves quickly on the meat, taking little time to chew in case another fiercer or stronger predator drove them from their meal. Also, the more dominant and greedy the individual wolf was, the better the chance of survival. Literally, they "wolfed down" their food. They would then seek out a safe retreat in which to rest and digest their food and often would not need to eat again for two or three days. Their stomachs were adapted to accept hastily gulped, chunky food and then to digest it slowly. Although our pet dogs today are civilized versions of this ancestor, their digestive tracts have not changed all that much, and their eating patterns remain very similar to the way they were in the wild. Some very secure pet dogs do eat slowly, but this is the exception rather than the rule.

Because pet owners tend to project human characteristics onto their animals, they may interpret the dog's hasty eating habits as joyless. Human pleasure in eating is evidenced by slow chewing while savoring the taste and texture of a food. Such chewing activity does not happen in dogs; in fact, there exists a fundamental biological difference between the mechanisms of eating in humans and dogs. Human saliva contains an enzyme called amylase, which digests starch, and to allow this enzyme to start working, humans need to chew their food into smaller particles. This is an instinctive process which stimulates the taste and smell nerves, thereby increasing the production of saliva and gastric (stomach) digestive juices. In people, well-chewed food becomes well lubricated and easier to swallow and is therefore more readily acted upon by the gastric juices. The saliva of dogs does not contain digestive enzymes and functions only as a lubricant to aid swallowing, so that chewing is not as necessary in dogs as it is in people.

Interestingly, many present-day primitive tribes that depend on hunting eat by gorging themselves when a kill is made and then not eating again for up to a week. The average American would have extreme difficulty adapting to this feeding pattern, but domestic dogs appear to be able to adjust to it quite readily. Studies show that many domestic dogs that have gone feral (wild) have quickly reverted to the feeding patterns of their ancient wild ancestors.

FIBER AND GRASS EATING

There is a lot of emphasis on the need for fiber in the human diet, and dogs need fiber in their diets for the same reasons that people do. Fiber in the diet has the following benefits and effects:

1. It regulates the digestive system by providing bulk, which aids in moving food through the system.

2. It helps to absorb water from the digestive tract, which results in larger and more acceptably formed stools.

3. It provides stimulation of the intestinal muscles and keeps them in good tone.

4. It decreases the time it takes food to pass through the digestive tract, which, together with the bulkier stools, may lower the risk of colon cancer by reducing the exposure time of the bowel wall to naturally occurring colon carcinogens.

5. It is useful in filling out diets used in weight reduction, because it has no food value.

All commercial dog foods that have cereal in their formula contain fiber, and I do not know of any commercial dog food produced in the United States today that does not contain some cereal.

We do not know why dogs eat grass. This may actually be to fill a need for fiber, although this has not been confirmed scientifically. Eating grass could also fill a nutritional need, but even healthy, well-nourished dogs eat grass, so investigations in this area have not been fruitful. There is no doubt that dogs frequently vomit after eating grass, and logically it has been assumed that they eat the grass to induce vomiting because of an upset stomach. Most dogs can vomit voluntarily, so this explanation is also less than satisfactory. Wolves, the ancestor of the dog, ate the stomach contents of their kills, most of which were grass-eating animals—so perhaps the answer is here, and this was their fiber source or filled some other nutritional need we still do not understand. Until we know more about it, grass eating should not be discouraged in dogs.

TABLE SCRAPS

Veterinarians are frequently asked if it is all right to feed a dog table scraps, and one expert on canine nutrition always answers this question like this: "What would you do with these table scraps if you did not own a dog?" If the answer is "save them for another meal," the scraps are probably fine for the dog. If the scraps would go into the garbage, then that's more than likely what they are, and feeding a dog garbage is not of much nutritional value.

There are advantages and disadvantages to feeding dogs table scraps, the former being that food is not being wasted in a world where protein is scarce and waste is inexcusable; and mixed with the dog's basic diet of commercial dog food, scraps may make the food more palatable, thereby encouraging the dog to eat it. The disadvantages are: table scraps are often high in fats and carbohydrates, supplying lots of empty calories but not much balanced nutrition, and may, for the same reason lead to obesity; the dog may develop the bad habit of begging at the dining table; the dog may soon refuse to eat the balanced commercial dog food which should be its basic diet; the dog may pick out and eat only the scraps, if they are mixed with its regular food; and if scraps make up more than 10% of the dog's diet, the balanced dog food will no longer be eaten in sufficient quantity to remain balanced and supply all the dog's nutritional needs.

Each dog owner must decide if any of the disadvantages are severe enough to create problems with the dog. If not, then 10% of the diet as table scraps is acceptable and palliates the owner's conscience that food is not being wasted. It is probably best to make table scraps treats rather than part of the dog's daily diet.

CAT FOOD FOR DOGS

The nutritional requirements of cats are very different from those of dogs, and for this reason commercial cat foods should not be fed to dogs, even though they like it, except as an occasional treat. Cats require a higher protein content in their foods than dogs and most of this protein for cats needs to come from meat to meet their nutritional requirements. Dogs can thrive on food without any animal protein, utilizing plant proteins to meet their needs.

The high cost of meat protein, together with the pressure of world opinion that feeding meat protein (which is in short supply in many Third World countries) to dogs is wasteful, has forced pet food manufacturers to formulate dog foods consisting mostly of plant protein. Also, all-meat diets can lead to nutritional deficiencies in dogs, and because of their richness often cause diarrhea.

Despite all this sensible reasoning, the fact remains that dogs still prefer meat protein to plant protein—and this explains why they like cat food so much. Used as a treat, cat food is acceptable, but if it is fed in larger quantities it provides an excess of protein that can damage the kidneys. The dog may also acquire a taste for canned cat food and refuse to eat its own food.

SNACKS AND OTHER FOODS FOR DOGS

If you want to give a dog a snack or a treat, the best choice is a commercial product marketed for such purposes, as most are nutritionally complete and will not create a nutritional imbalance. A brief outline follows of other foods which can be fed to dogs, and foods which should be avoided. If a dog is being fed a commercial dog food, none of these additional foods should make up more than 10% of the diet.

Milk. Milk is an excellent source of calcium, protein, and many vitamins, and can be fed to dogs in reasonable quantities. The only contraindications are if it causes diarrhea; if the dog is already overweight; or if gastrointestinal or skin symptoms due to a milk allergy occur.

Raw meat. Meat is more nutritious if fed raw to a dog, but most dogs today prefer their meat cooked. Pork, rabbit, and wild animal meat should be well cooked to avoid the danger of parasite transmission.

Vegetables. Dogs do not digest vegetables very well unless they are cooked. Most vegetables can be fed to dogs (if they will eat them), although green leaf vegetables are of little value to them nutritionally.

Fish. Fish is an excellent source of protein for a dog. It should be cooked to avoid parasite transmission, and the bones should be removed.

Eggs. Eggs are one of the best sources of protein available. One or two eggs a week, cooked, are recommended.

Cheese. Cheese is also an excellent source of protein and of fat, but is a somewhat expensive food for dogs.

Liver. Liver supplies valuable proteins, fats, carbohydrates, vitamins, and minerals and is an excellent food, particularly for sick or weak dogs. It is more nutritious raw, but most dogs will only accept it if it is cooked.

Fats and oils. Fats and oils help to maintain a healthy skin and haircoat in a dog. Some dry dog foods are low in fat, so if a dog's skin is dry and flaky, give him one tablespoon of bacon fat or corn oil per pound of dry food, per day. Beef fat is also useful as a source of extra energy in the diet, but it will not supply adequately the essential fatty acids if they are deficient (bacon fat and corn oil do supply these).

Chocolate. Chocolate should not be fed because it contains theobromine, and this is quite toxic to dogs.

Candy and cake. Many dogs love these foods. The problem with feeding dogs these high-calorie foods is that the dog may not then eat enough of his dog food to be properly nourished. Too much sugar may cause digestive upsets, lead to obesity, or cause tooth cavities—problems humans are all too well aware of!

Onions and garlic. Many dog owners are convinced onions and even more so, garlic, get rid of or prevent worms and fleas. This has not been confirmed scientifically despite a number of investigations. Small quantities of either will not harm your dog, but they make close contact less pleasant!

Alcohol. There is no good reason to give a dog alcohol, but if used in moderation, it should not be harmful.

Fruits. Fruits are of very little value to the dog nutritionally, nor do dogs like them. For man, fruits are a source of vitamin C, but dogs synthesize their own vitamin C and do not need an outside source of supply.

Cereal grains. Cereal grains are good sources of protein and carbohydrates for dogs, and most dog foods are high in corn, soybean, or wheat.

Bread. Bread is a very good basic food and should be fed to dogs if you are going to throw it out. Don't overdo it, however, and don't use it if your dog is overweight.

Potatoes. Potatoes must be cooked for dogs to digest them. They can be used in place of other carbohydrates on occasion.

Spaghetti, noodles, macaroni, and rice. These are all excellent carbohydrate sources and are well liked by most dogs.

Brewer's yeast and wheat germ. These products are sources of many essential vitamins and are added to most commercial dog foods.

Bone meal. Bone meal contains calcium and phosphorus in the correct ratio for a dog, but it should not be used unless the dog is being fed extra meat. Add one-half ounce for every pound of meat added to the diet.

2
Parasites

Parasites are animals or insects that live upon (external) or within (internal) another living organism at whose expense they obtain nourishment and shelter. Parasites devour blood or damage tissues of their unwilling hosts, but contribute nothing in return. The vast majority of parasites cause damage to their hosts.

Discussion will focus first on internal parasites.

INTERNAL PARASITES

Although there are many internal parasites that infect dogs, the emphasis here is on roundworms, tapeworms, and hookworms, as they are the most frequently encountered in pet dogs.

The symptoms of internal parasites in dogs will depend on the location of the parasite. Intestinal parasites cause digestive problems, most commonly diarrhea, but many also utilize the food eaten by the host and thereby weaken the animal by depriving it of essential nutrients. Parasites in the respiratory tract cause coughing. Many parasites destroy blood, which results in anemia and can lead to death if the blood loss is severe. Specific signs of each type of internal parasite are hard to define, as they depend on the organ(s) affected and the severity of the infection. The most common sign of parasitism in dogs is an overall unhealthy condition.

Parasites weaken an animal and lower its resistance to disease. They also often carry bacterial and viral infections with them, so they not only open the way for disease but often transport it as well. The age of the animal, its state of health, and the number of parasites all determine the effects the parasite will have on the host animal. Young animals are most susceptible, followed by poorly nourished, sick, and old animals. A healthy, well-nourished animal should have sufficient natural defenses against parasites unless the exposure is overwhelming.

Diagnosis of Internal Parasites

The most universal sign of internal parasitism in dogs is a general "unthrifty" or unwell condition. The haircoat may be thin and rough, and bowel movements may be abnormal. Frequently, the symptoms are nonspecific and for this reason, some or all of the following laboratory tests are required to make an accurate diagnosis:

1. *Stool examination.* Gross examination of the dog's stool can be used to diagnose most species of tapeworm as the segments can often be seen in the stool. While whole worms are seldom seen in the stool, they may occasionally be observed in massive infections of roundworms in puppies.

2. *Vomitus examination.* Stomach worms, and sometimes roundworms and tapeworms, may be vomited; they can then be identified by their appearance.

3. *Fecal analysis.* Most worms that infect dogs can be diagnosed from a fecal analysis. A small stool sample is adequate, and should be refrigerated if there is a delay in getting it to your veterinary hospital. Dog owners can pick up special containers and get instructions on how to obtain this sample prior to collection if they suspect their dogs have worms. Following dilution and centrifugation, examination under a high-powered microscope will reveal the eggs and/or larvae of the adult worms, which can then be identified.

4. *Blood tests.* Special blood tests are required to identify blood parasites and heartworms.

5. *Urine analysis.* Bladder and kidney worms are diagnosed by identifying the eggs microscopically in the urine.

6. *Biopsy.* Examination of infected tissue samples may be required to diagnose toxoplasmosis and other parasites which invade internal body organs.

Treatment of Internal Parasites

There are many different treatments available for controlling internal parasites; most are done with drugs; a few are surgical.

All worming medications are dangerous drugs, and all are potentially toxic to the dog. Their effective use depends on giving a sufficient dose to kill the worms without endangering the dog's life. Effective over-the-counter drugs are available for treating roundworms in dogs, but not for other internal parasites. Your veterinarian must consider many factors before worming a dog. The decision whether to do the worming in a hospital or at home is influenced by such factors as:

1. The type of parasite.
2. The relative danger of the medication.
3. The possible need for an enema.
4. The dog's age and condition.
5. The dog's medical history.
6. The ability of the owner to medicate the dog correctly and without getting bitten.
7. The likelihood of the owner's being upset if such side reactions as vomiting or diarrhea occur or masses of worms are passed.
8. Most importantly, the owner's ability to judge if the dog suffers a real toxic reaction and should be taken to the veterinary hospital for treatment.

New worming products, in which the toxic side effects such as vomiting and diarrhea are being reduced and the worms are predigested prior to evacuation, are continually being developed. This makes worming less dangerous and less messy, and has allowed veterinarians to dispense worming medications for home use. However, directions concerning dosage, fasting, and observation of the dog must be closely followed to avoid complications and to ensure effective treatment.

For most worms, two wormings ten to fourteen days apart are recommended. Some internal parasites require daily and/or long-term medication for control. For a few, fortunately rare, internal parasites, there are no treatments or the treatments are only partially effective.

Preventing Infection and Reinfection

Many veterinary clients are frustrated because their dogs so frequently become reinfected with worms following worming. Some blame their veterinarian for not doing a thorough job. If worms reappear in less than a month, it is likely that they were not all eliminated by the worming. This is often the case with tapeworms, as they are difficult to dislodge from the intestinal wall and may shed only their bodies, while the head remains, allowing regrowth. If the worms appear again in two to three months, then reinfection is more likely. Many dog owners do not realize that worming a dog is not enough; preventive measures against reinfection, such as the following, must be taken:

Control of external parasites. Since fleas, lice, and ticks are the intermediate hosts for many internal parasites in dogs, it is essential to use insecticides to eliminate them or a dog will be quickly reinfected.

Proper sanitation. If reinfection can come from contact with stools infected by such parasites as roundworms and hookworms, daily removal of the stool and washing down the area are essential. Sunlight, dryness, and heat destroy most worms, eggs, and larvae; there are products available to spray on dog runs or areas where dogs defecate which will kill the larvae. Because rodents and cockroaches are also sources of internal parasite infection for dogs, they must be controlled to prevent reinfection. Cleanliness and good housekeeping are the most important—and most neglected—preventive measures in parasite control in dogs.

Care in feeding meat and fish. Dogs should not be allowed to eat their prey if they hunt. While raw beef is usually safe when bought in a supermarket, it can never be 100% guaranteed parasite-free; raw fish should not be fed to dogs. Pork, of course, should never be fed raw to pets or people because of the danger of trichinosis. The best prevention is to cook all meat and fish well.

Attention to nutrition. Healthy, well-fed dogs can build up immunity to many internal parasites. Weak, undernourished dogs, and particularly puppies, will fall victim to every parasite to which they are exposed.

Care of breeding dogs. All dogs used for breeding should be routinely wormed for roundworms prior to mating, and checked for other internal parasites and wormed if infected.

Adherence to routine examination schedule. All puppies should be checked for worms when they are six weeks old, earlier if they show signs of worms. Routine roundworming is recommended for all puppies, starting as early as two weeks of age if infections are suspected. Adult dogs should have a fecal analysis done once a year. Owners should check their dog's stools for signs of tapeworms.

Attention to health in a multi-dog household. If one dog in a multi-dog household is found to be infected with worms, then all the other dogs should be checked or routinely wormed also. Whenever a new dog is introduced into a household, it should be isolated from the other dogs until it has been checked by a veterinarian for signs of disease or parasite infection. Some of the worms which infect dogs can also infect cats, so the same checking process will be required if there are cats in the household.

Roundworms

Toxocara canis and *Toxascaris leonina* are the round-worms most commonly occurring in dogs. Most puppies, as previously mentioned, are born already infected. The adult worms are from 2 to 6 inches long and 1/16 inch wide; the males are smaller than the females. They live free in the intestines of the infected dog.

The life cycle of *Toxocara canis* is complex, but knowledge of it will help to explain why most puppies are born infected. The female worms produce eggs which pass out in the dog's stool, but it may take up to two weeks before larvae develop within the eggs, which then become infective. (The larva is a development stage of a parasite; for example, the caterpillar is the larva of a butterfly.) There are six possible modes of roundworm infection in dogs:

1. *Puppies.* If infective eggs are eaten by a puppy less than five weeks old, the larvae migrate through the liver and lungs and back to the intestines, where they mature into round-worms.

2. *Puppies and adult dogs.* If the infective eggs are eaten by a puppy over five weeks old or by an adult dog, the larvae migrate through the body where they become encysted (en-

Roundworms (Life-sized)

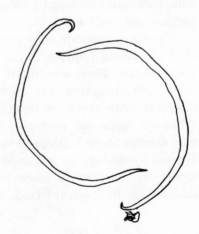

closed in a sac) in the tissues and remain; the cycle is then incomplete and no intestinal worms result.

3. *Puppies.* If a dog harboring encysted larvae becomes pregnant, the larvae again become active and enter the fetus; this is how puppies are born already infected. The larvae in the fetus remain in the liver and lungs, but as soon as the pups are born, the larvae escape from the lungs, are coughed up and swallowed; they mature in about three weeks in the intestines of the puppies.

4. *Puppies.* Larvae can be passed to the puppies in the mother's milk.

5. *Adult dogs.* Infective eggs can be consumed by other hosts, such as chickens, mice, earthworms, etc.; they do not mature in these hosts, however, but remain in a resting stage. If a dog consumes any of these intermediate hosts harboring larvae, adult roundworms will develop in the intestines.

6. *Mother dogs.* The female dog may also become infected with adult intestinal roundworms if her puppies are infected.

The life cycle of *Toxascaris leonina* is more direct: the larvae from the eggs enter the intestinal wall for a few weeks and then return to the intestines and mature as worms in about forty-five days. These larvae do not migrate and are not, therefore, transmitted prenatally. Dogs can also be infected with *Toxascaris leonina* by eating other hosts, such as mice, cockroaches, and earthworms.

SYMPTOMS Roundworms can cause severe illness, particularly in young puppies. These worms rob the puppies of nourishment. They also interfere with the digestive processes, often resulting in vomiting and diarrhea and, in heavy infections, can result in bowel obstruction or perforation. When the larvae are migrating through the liver and lungs, they damage these organs, and signs of anemia and respiratory distress (coughing) are apparent. Bronchitis and even pneumonia are not unusual consequences of heavy roundworm infections in puppies. Infected puppies are weak, restless, cry a lot, are thin with pot bellies, fail to thrive, and have dull haircoats and eyes. Adult dogs are not as severely affected, but do tend to look unwell, with dull haircoats.

DIAGNOSIS Your veterinarian can diagnose roundworms by testing a fecal sample and identifying the worm eggs under the microscope. Worms can sometimes be seen in the stool or may even be vomited in heavy infections. It is best to assume that all puppies are infected and to worm them routinely.

TREATMENT Many drugs are available from veterinarians for controlling roundworms, and piperazine, the roundworm medication sold by pet stores, is effective. If you decide to worm the puppies with over-the-counter medications, dosage and directions must be followed carefully. The "if some is good, more is better" approach to treatment has caused severe illness and even fatalities in puppies. Your veterinarian can do these wormings for you, and this is advisable if the puppies are unwell. It is recommended that the stools be checked after a full course of worming treatments to be sure the worms have been eliminated. Yearly fecal testing is a good idea if your dog is continually exposed to reinfection.

PREVENTION Roundworm eggs are very resistant to destruction, and can survive freezing and most disinfectants. Sunlight and dryness destroy them. To prevent infection, or reinfection, good sanitation is important, and this includes control of rodents and cockroaches.

Unfortunately, there is no effective drug available to rid a female dog of encysted larvae—which is why success in eliminating roundworms in dogs has not been achieved. Experimentally, breeding females have been freed of infection, but the treatments are as yet too difficult for routine application.

Tapeworms

The most common tapeworm infecting dogs is *Dipylidium caninum*, also referred to as the flea tapeworm. These worms can reach 20 inches in length. An understanding of the life cycle of the tapeworm is helpful in preventing reinfection.

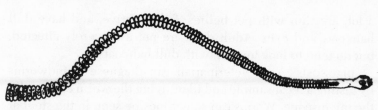

Flea Tapeworm (Life-sized)

All tapeworms in dogs require an intermediate host, and for *Dipylidium* it is the flea. The tapeworm eggs are enclosed in end segments of the worm's body that are expelled in an infected dog's stool. These are then eaten by flea larvae, hatched from flea eggs. When these larvae mature into fleas and the dog swallows one, the tapeworm is released from the flea by the digestive juices, and attaches itself to the dog's intestinal wall. There it grows, eating some of the dog's food; upon reaching maturity, it begins to pass segments filled with eggs, thus completing the life cycle.

SYMPTOMS   These tapeworms do not cause a lot of harm to the dog. An increase in appetite is often noted, and there may be some local damage to the intestines where the worms attach with hooklike projections, which can sometimes lead to digestive upsets such as diarrhea. Itching of the anus from the segments crawling out can lead to the dog biting this area or scooting its hind end along the ground.

DIAGNOSIS   Your veterinarian can diagnose tapeworms by testing a fecal sample for the end segments of the worm's body, which break off and are passed out in the dog's stool. These segments contain pouches of eggs and when fresh in the stool are about ¼ to ½ inch long, cucumber-shaped, pinkish-white, and moving. When the segments dry out, they look like grains of rice and can often be seen stuck to the dog's hair around the anus. The dog cannot be directly infected by eating these segments.

TREATMENT   Tapeworm medication should be available only through a veterinarian, as all these products are potent drugs and not without hazardous side effects (unlike some of the roundworm medications). While many veterinarians dispense these medications for the dog owner to use at home, it is essential that all directions concerning fasting and dosages be followed carefully. Some dog owners prefer to have the veterinarian do the worming for tapeworms; this has certain advantages, but can be more expensive. Dogs often vomit worming medications before they have been effective, and this, of course, is more readily observed in the hospital environment. With the older, more hazardous, tapeworm medications the worms were expelled and could be checked to be sure the head, as well as the body, was dislodged. Many of the newer—and safer—medications cause the worms to break up before being expelled, and it is not possible to determine immediately if the worming was successful.

Despite many effective worming medications, tapeworms are difficult to destroy completely. If the worm segments reappear in the stool in less than a month, the tapeworm head was probably not dislodged, and the worm has grown again.

PREVENTION The only way to prevent infection and reinfection is to control fleas (*see* section later in this chapter). Because it is extremely difficult to keep a dog and a dog's environment completely free of fleas, reinfection is quite common. In temperate zones, which are warm all year, recurrence of tapeworm infection is very common, not only because fleas are difficult to control, but also because many of the insecticides available are no longer effective against fleas.

OTHER TAPEWORMS IN DOGS Other common tapeworms in dogs are from the *Taenia* species; the intermediate hosts are numerous and include rabbits, squirrels, rats and other rodents; sheep, goats, pigs, cattle, and even humans. There is also a dog tapeworm in which fish are the intermediate hosts. Your veterinarian can determine which tapeworm a dog has by examining the segments, or, if these are not seen, then by microscopic examination of the eggs in a fecal sample. The signs, diagnosis, and treatment are the same as for *Dipylid-*

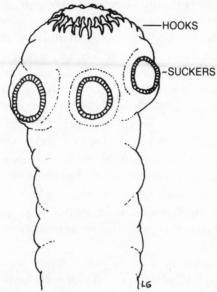

Taenia Tapeworm Head (Enlarged)

ium. Prevention involves not allowing the dog to consume the intermediate hosts.

Hookworms

There are three species of hookworms in dogs in the United States—*Ancylostoma caninum, A. brasiliense,* and *Unicinaria stenocephala.* These worms are small and thread-like, ¼ to ¾ inch long. The adult worms live in the intestines, where they hook on to the intestine wall—hence the name "hookworm." These worms are prevalent in warm, moist areas.

The female hookworm produces eggs, which pass out in the dog's stool. In about one week the larvae develop from these eggs and cause infection by being eaten by a dog, or by penetrating a dog's skin. In a few weeks the larvae develop into worms in the dog's intestine. Larvae that penetrate the skin and sometimes even those that are eaten migrate throughout the dog's body, and as a result, puppies can be infected while still in the uterus, or via the mother's milk.

SYMPTOMS   Hookworms suck blood from the intestinal wall, secreting an anticoagulant from their mouths to keep the blood flowing. This leads to severe blood loss and bloody diarrhea. Adult dogs will be anemic, weak, and thin, and puppies may die before any signs of infection are seen. The larvae can cause damage to other body tissues during migration and the most obvious signs of such damage are in the lungs— bronchitis or pneumonia. The skin can also show signs of irritation, especially the feet, where the larvae penetrate.

DIAGNOSIS   Diagnosis of hookworm infection is made by clinical signs and by microscopic identification of the eggs in a fecal sample.

TREATMENT   Some dogs may require blood transfusions and other supportive hospital care before worming can be undertaken. There are a number of oral drugs that destroy the adult worms; one drug is given by injection. A second worming is required in two weeks to kill any larvae that may have been in the migratory stage at the first worming. A high protein diet, iron, and vitamins are also recommended to help the dog quickly replenish the blood lost from its body.

PREVENTION   In areas of high infection, a preventive medication can be given daily in the food. There is also a promising vaccine available. Prevention of infection can be accomplished by good sanitation. In general, sunlight and dryness kill the larvae, and there are a number of products available for killing the larvae in areas where control is difficult.

Other Internal Parasites in Dogs

Whipworms. These are small, thin worms 2 to 3 inches long, which live in the cecum (large intestines) and colon of the dog. Often they cause no symptoms, but can cause diarrhea and weight loss. Diagnosis is made by identification of the eggs microscopically in a fecal sample. There is an effective drug for treatment available.

Stomach worms. These are similar to roundworms, but live in the stomach rather than the intestines; and they attach to the wall of the stomach. They cause gastritis or inflammation of the stomach, which may lead to vomiting. Drug treatment is effective. Cockroaches and beetles are thought to be involved in the life cycle of these worms.

Threadworms. These are very small worms, about ⅙ inch long, from the *Strongyloides* species. They locate in the intestines and cause diarrhea, which may be bloody. The larvae can penetrate the skin, causing a dermatitis. Drug treatment is possible, but not always successful.

Esophageal worms. These worms are 1 to 3 inches long and live in the walls of the esophagus; they may also locate in other areas of the body. They occur mostly in the southern United States. They cause vomiting, weakness, emaciation, and difficulty in swallowing. Treatment is difficult and seldom successful.

Kidney worms. These are very large worms, up to 3 feet in length and ¼ inch thick. They destroy the kidney, where they locate, and eventually lead to kidney failure. Treatment is by surgical removal.

Bladder worms. These worms locate in the bladder and are ½ to 2 inches long. They damage the bladder and there is no known treatment. Fortunately, they are rare in dogs.

Lungworms. These worms are about 1 inch long, and because of their location, they cause coughing and lung irritation. Treatment is difficult and only partially successful.

Flukes. These are small, ¼-inch-long parasites which locate in the liver and lungs of dogs, causing disease in these organs. Most are transmitted by infected raw fish. Treatment is not satisfactory. A disease known as salmon poisoning, which causes severe illness and bloody diarrhea in dogs, is caused by an organism which is carried by flukes and infects salmon and trout. It is prevalent in the Pacific Northwest. The disease can be avoided by cooking fish or deep freezing.

Eye worms. These are ½-inch-long worms which infect the eyes of dogs. They are transmitted by flies, are relatively common in California, and can be removed surgically.

Blood parasites. There are a number of blood parasites which infect dogs, but the most common is *Hemobartonella,* a microscopic parasite which attacks red blood cells. Response to treatment is usually good in the early stages of the disease.

Protozoa. Protozoa are unicellular, microscopic organisms. Coccidiosis, giardiasis, and amebiasis are protozoan diseases in dogs which cause diarrhea, poor appetite, and weakness. These are intestinal diseases and most respond well to treatment.

Toxoplasmosis. This is another protozoan disease which can affect many organs of the body. The symptoms relate to the affected area. Treatment is possible, depending on the area of infection.

Heartworms. (*See* Chapter 8, The Heart; Heartworm Disease.)

EXTERNAL PARASITES

Like internal parasites, external parasites—fleas, lice, ticks, mites, and flies—are commonly encountered in dogs. They cause multiple problems, such as:

- Skin irritation, which leads to scratching and self-inflicted injury.
- Transmission of many serious diseases.
- Transmission of tapeworms (fleas and lice).
- Serious skin diseases.
- Anemia.

Fleas

Fleas are the most widespread of all external parasites of dogs. They are small, flat, black, fast-moving, jumping insects, about ⅛ inch long; they are readily visible to the naked eye. There are over 1,400 species of fleas, but those which commonly cause problems for pet owners are: *Ctenocephalides canis*—the dog flea; *C. felis*—the cat flea; *Echnidophaga gallinacea*—the sticktight flea of poultry; and *Pulex irritans*—the human flea. Each of these species tends to stay on its own host, but will attack other hosts if deprived of its preferred host. However, today's dog owner really need worry about only one type of flea—the cat flea. Human and dog fleas are seldom seen today.

Flea bites cause extreme irritation and many dogs are allergic to flea saliva, which can result in severe skin problems (*see* Chapter 4, The Skin; Allergic Skin Diseases). Fleas suck blood from their host, and this can lead to anemia in heavy infestations and in young or debilitated dogs. They also transmit many bacterial, viral, and parasitic diseases, and are the intermediate hosts for the flea-transmitted tapeworm.

Fleas thrive in warm moist climates, are readily destroyed by cold or dryness. As a result, they are not as severe a problem in the colder or desert regions of the United States, but tend to be a year-round problem in the more temperate zones, such as California and Florida. An understanding of the life cycle of the flea is helpful in choosing methods of control.

There are four stages to the life cycle of the dog flea: the egg, larva, pupa, and adult. The time for completion of the full life cycle varies from two weeks to one-and-a-half years, and an adult flea can live up to two years under laboratory conditions, although the average life span is three to four weeks for males, and six to nine weeks for females on a dog. These wide variations are affected by temperature, humidity, food availability, and other environmental factors.

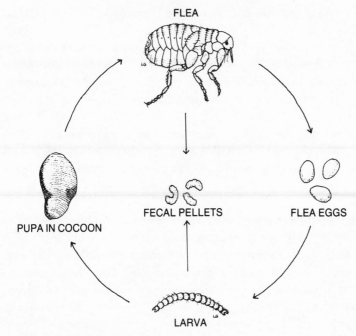

FLEA

FECAL PELLETS

FLEA EGGS

PUPA IN COCOON

LARVA

Life Cycle of the Dog Flea

Adult fleas. Adult fleas live on a dog which can support up to 100 fleas a week, and both the male and female fleas require a blood meal before they mate. The female flea lays up to twenty eggs a day, and over her lifetime can lay hundreds of eggs. Since fleas do not survive more than one month if separated from their host, they will seek out any warm-blooded animal if their host is unavailable or has more fleas than it can support—which explains why people start getting bitten when the infestations are heavy. After a blood meal, fleas pass fecal pellets (stool), which are made up of partially digested blood. These fecal pellets look like grains of pepper and if you wet them they dissolve into a reddish fluid.

Eggs. Flea eggs are visible to the naked eye as tiny, egg-shaped, white specks. They are laid on the dog and fall off;

occasionally, if the flea leaves the dog, they are deposited in other areas.

Dogs infested with fleas leave a salt-and-pepper debris of eggs and fecal pellets wherever they lie. (Veterinarians often point out this debris falling off a dog on the examining table to clients who are quite positive that their dog has no fleas!)

Larvae. The eggs hatch in a few days and release flea larvae, which look like small worms, barely visible to the naked eye. They feed on fecal pellets and any other available food or organic debris. These larvae pass through two more larval stages over the next few months. They are not often seen by dog owners as they do not live on the dog, but tend instead to locate in floor cracks, rugs, or damp areas.

Pupae. The third-stage larvae spin a cocoon and, like caterpillars, they pupate or metamorphose. They emerge as an adult flea when the temperature is about 80 degrees Fahrenheit and the humidity is 80%; or from pressure, such as being stepped on. They immediately seek a host to feed and breed on.

As a result of this pressure sensitivity pet owners who return from vacation before picking up their boarding pets may be immediately attacked by fleas desperate for their first meal. The same thing often occurs when someone rents premises in which a pet resided and moves in without a pet. Given a choice, these fleas will attack a dog or cat—but humans will do if nothing else is available! When your dog goes crazy running around the house upon return from a vacation or absence, it's being driven mad by flea bites, and not with delight at getting home again!

FLEA CONTROL   Flea control is more difficult today than in the past because many of the most effective insecticides have been removed from the market due to environmental pollution problems. Fleas readily build up resistance to the available insecticides and are no longer affected by them. Since the main approach to flea control is to break the flea life cycle, one must kill the fleas and get rid of the eggs, larvae, and pupae. This is not an easy task, nor is there any one method of control that will eradicate fleas. Rather, one must take several steps to control fleas, and keep them up throughout the flea season, which can be all year-round in some areas. Contrary to what is occasionally seen in the press, ultrasound devices are not effective in flea control. The following control measures, however, *are* recommended:

Flea sprays, powders, shampoos, and dips. Weekly washing with insecticidal shampoos or the use of flea dips is one of the most effective methods of controlling fleas on dogs. Alternatively, weekly spraying or powdering with flea-control insecticides may be used. Use fresh products and follow directions carefully. If the fleas are not being killed, try another product, and ask your veterinarian for advice, since some insecticides will be more effective in your area than others. Most veterinarians dispense flea-control products, and can show and advise dog owners how to use them effectively and safely. Insecticides are poisonous, but used according to directions, their benefits far outweigh their disadvantage, and flea control is essential for the health and comfort of the dog and all members of the household.

Flea collars. Flea collars are effective in controlling fleas on dogs in areas where the problem is seasonal and not severe. They are only partially effective in areas of heavy infestations. They must be used according to directions and should not be used if other insecticides are being applied to the dog, except under veterinary advice.

Fumigation. Combined with methods of flea control on the dog, fumigation is the best method of eliminating fleas from the dog's environment. An exterminating service can be used to spray inside and outside the house every few months if necessary, or you can do the interior extermination yourself, using insecticidal sprays or aerosol foggers sold by veterinarians, hardware stores, and pet stores. Most garden insect-control products will kill fleas if sprayed around the outside of the house or in outside areas the dog frequents. Do not, however, use such products inside the house. Do not use any fumigation products on the dog or the dog's bedding.

Vacuuming and area cleaning. Floors should be vacuumed frequently, with special attention paid to areas where the dog lies. Dog flea sprays or powders should be used on the dog's bedding or areas it frequents.

Combing. Many dog owners use a special flea comb to remove fleas from their dog. While this is certainly helpful, it is very time-consuming and will not control a flea problem by itself.

Flea control oral medications. A veterinarian can dispense tablets and liquids that control fleas. These are systemic insecticides and are given to the dog by mouth. They are rapidly absorbed and distributed throughout the body tissues and bloodstream. Fleas and other biting insects are killed when they ingest the drug on biting the dog. If used early in the flea season and for limited periods of time, these products can be safe and effective, but they do require veterinary supervision. Dogs taking these products must not be exposed to other insecticides. (*See* Flea Control Medications, later in this chapter, for further information on these products.)

STICKTIGHT FLEAS Although these are fleas of poultry, they are sometimes seen on dogs. They are smaller than dog or cat fleas and they attach themselves to the dog's skin, most commonly on the face. They then lay eggs under the skin, which leads to intense irritation. They can be removed with tweezers, or killed with the careful use of flea sprays.

Ticks

Ticks are small, dark, crawling insects with eight legs; they are usually ⅛ to ¼ inch long. (The female can swell up to ½ inch when engorged with blood.) There are a number of ticks which attack dogs, but only three are encountered with any frequency. Two are hard-bodied ticks, *Dermacentor variabilis*—American dog tick, and *Rhipicephalus sanguineus*—

brown dog tick; and one is soft-bodied, *Otobius megnini*—
spinose ear tick.

Ticks cause local irritation at the point of attachment; they
also carry a number of diseases. The American dog tick is
found from east of the Rocky Mountains to the West Coast.
This tick carries Rocky Mountain spotted fever, which can be
serious in humans. Another serious disease, tick paralysis, is
seen occasionally in humans and dogs and is caused by a
neurotoxin produced by the feeding female tick. The brown
dog tick is widely distributed throughout the United States
and Canada. Hard ticks are mostly a problem in rural areas,
particularly in wooded and mountainous terrains. Spinose ear
ticks are found in dry regions of the southwestern U.S.

All ticks have similar life cycles. Adult ticks attack dogs as
they walk through vegetation, attaching themselves to the dog
with their mouth parts and sucking blood. The ticks mate on
the dog, and the female continues to engorge for about ten
days, after which she drops off and lays up to 6,000 eggs over
the next few weeks. The adults die at this point. In about one
month, the six-legged larval ticks emerge from the eggs and
attach themselves to small mammals to feed for a few days.
They then drop off and are transformed into eight-legged
nymphs over the next month. The nymphs then attach themselves to small mammals for a meal, drop off, and become
adults in one to nine months. The life cycle time period is
variable and depends on the temperature, humidity, and other

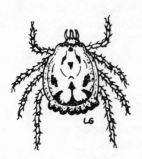

Hard-bodied Dog Tick (Enlarged)

environmental conditions; under optimum conditions, it can be completed in as little as three months.

While most ticks feed on a variety of mammals, the brown dog tick can remain on the dog for all stages of its life cycle, and for this reason it is more difficult to control. Only the larvae and nymphs of the spinose ear tick attack dogs, and as the name suggests, they locate in the ear—the adults do not feed.

TICK CONTROL   Tick control is similar to flea control, but as ticks are more resistant to insecticides, in heavily infested areas some will always manage to attach, even with the most intensive preventive measures. Dog owners can remove adult ticks by grasping them close to their skin attachment with fingernails or tweezers, and pulling gently until the tick lets go. No attempt to burn them off with a cigarette should be made, or the head will remain embedded and may lead to an abscess.

Application of insecticides to ticks will sometimes make them let go, but is not always successful—and this method poses some hazard of poisoning and pain to the dog if the insecticide comes in contact with the skin wound, particularly when removing a lot of ticks. Flea dips and sprays will kill ticks in a few days, but hand removal is recommended daily in tick problem areas. Insecticidal ear solutions effectively kill the spinose ear ticks. Clearing brush, spraying with insecticides, and keeping dogs out of tick-infested areas will, of course, keep the problem to a minimum. Since ticks are not as species-specific as other insects and will attack man, humans may need to take precautions in tick-infested areas.

Lice

Lice are small, about ⅙ inch, flat, fast-moving, almost colorless insects. There are two types of lice: biting and sucking. They spend their entire lives on the dog and only live a few hours off the animal.

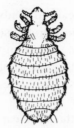

Dog Louse (Enlarged)

While lice are seldom a problem in dogs if they and their quarters are kept clean, lice can cause intense irritation and itching. Most of the damage is from self-inflicted trauma from scratching, even to the point of bleeding. This can lead to anemia or infected wounds. Lice can also transmit a number of diseases.

The life cycle of lice, from egg, through four nymph stages, to adult takes about thirty days. The adults live about one month. The eggs attach to the hairs and are commonly referred to as nits. They can readily be seen with a magnifying glass or even with the naked eye if the haircoat of the dog is closely examined. The adults are difficult to see.

LICE CONTROL   Control is the same as for fleas. Lice are species-specific and those of the dog are not readily contagious to humans; humans have their own species of lice to contend with.

Ear Mites (*See* Chapter 6, The Ears; External Ear Disease: Ear Mites.)

Mange Mites (*See* Chapter 4, The Skin; Parasitic Skin Diseases.)

Fly Problems

Flies cause two main problems in dogs: One is caused by biting flies, and the other by flies which lay their eggs in flesh wounds.

Biting Flies. Dogs are often troubled by stable flies, which, while similar in appearance to houseflies, have one important difference: They bite the skin of humans and animals in order to suck blood. As their name implies, these flies are most abundant around stables. The life cycle, from egg to adult, is about 3 weeks.

These flies usually attack the ears and face of the dog. Not only are they very annoying, but their biting can transmit disease and result in wound infections.

FLY CONTROL   Ordinary fly repellents should be applied daily, or as often as necessary, to the affected skin areas to prevent further bites. These products are available in drug stores, pet stores, and saddleries. The human insect repellents are safe to use on dogs. Your local veterinary hospital may also have such products available or can make recommendations. Try to keep the dog inside during the day, if possible. If severe bites have been sustained, a cortisone-antibiotic ointment should be applied to the wounds to aid healing and prevent infections. The source of the stable flies should be investigated, because such areas need to be sprayed with insecticides every few weeks to keep the fly populations under control.

Myiasis (Fly Maggots). Some fly species lay their eggs in the wounds of animals, and a condition known as *cutaneous myiasis* results. When the eggs hatch, usually within twenty-four hours, the emerging larvae, also called maggots, can be seen on close inspection of the wound.

The maggots feed on the discharges from wounds and on flesh. If wounds are left untended, serious infections and even fatalities can occur.

Surgical treatment is required in most cases in order to kill the maggots with a mild insecticide, remove them, and to clean and treat the wound. Since a wound filled with maggots is a most distressing sight for a dog owner and hazardous and painful for the dog, owners should treat and keep an eye on all skin injuries to prevent *cutaneous myiasis* from occurring.

INSECTICIDES

All insecticides are poisonous products, but if used according to directions, their advantages far outweigh their disadvantages. The ideal insecticide should kill the insect without risk to the animal or to the person applying it, and it should not leave residues in the environment, or in tissues, eggs, or milk. No present-day insecticide meets all these requirements, but some are certainly closer to this ideal than others. It is essential to use some sort of insecticidal control for fleas, ticks, and lice to ensure the health and comfort of dogs and all other members of the household.

The major types of insecticides used on dogs are:

Natural or Botanical

Popular today for flea control in dogs is the feeding of B-vitamins, garlic, or brewer's yeast. Eucalyptus leaves, walnut oil, and cedar bedding are also popular for direct-contact flea control. Studies have been done to test the effectiveness of these methods of control, and none of them has been found to affect the insect population on the dog. Despite these negative results, many dog owners claim these methods are effective, particularly for flea control.

Pyrethrin is a natural insecticide derived from the flowers of certain species of chrysanthemum, which quickly stuns insects upon contact when used on the dog. However, unless the insects are removed at once, they may recover, and for this reason pyrethrin is usually combined with a longer-acting insecticide to enhance its effectiveness. Though toxic to insects, it is not as toxic to mammals as some of the synthetic insecticides.

Rotenone is another natural insecticide, derived from the derris root. It is relatively safe and reasonably effective when used on the dog.

Chlorinated Hydrocarbons

These insecticides tend to persist in the environment, are very toxic to fish, and accumulate in the fatty tissues of humans and animals; they are excreted in milk. For this reason their use is no longer permitted for insect control on dogs.

These insecticides act on the central nervous system, and no specific antidote is available. Signs of toxic overdosage are episodes of violent excitement and convulsions, followed by depression.

The most commonly used chlorinated hydrocarbons were DDT, methoxychlor, lindane, chlordane, toxaphene, dieldrin, and aldrin.

Organophosphates and Carbamates

These two classes of insecticides are grouped together because their action, which paralyzes nerve endings, is similar. They are more toxic to animals and humans than chlorinated hydrocarbons, but they do not persist in the environment, and are therefore more ecologically acceptable today. Also, antidotes are available for treatment of overdosages.

Organophosphates are not used to any extent today, and in many instances are no longer available for use on dogs. Dichlorvos was popular in flea collars, and malathion in flea sprays. Ronnel is the least toxic of this group of insecticides.

The carbamate class of insecticides is used extensively for external parasite control in dogs today. The best known of this group is carbaryl.

Signs of overdosage from organophosphate and carbamate insecticides are muscle tremors, excessive salivation, eye watering, vomiting, diarrhea, and eventually paralysis of the respiratory muscles, leading to death.

Precautions in the Use of Insecticides

Some recommended precautions for the safe and effective use of insecticides are:

1. Follow directions carefully.
2. Do not overuse sprays; dog's coat should not be soaking wet.
3. Do not leave excessive amounts of powder on the dog; rub or brush it off following application.
4. Never use a flea collar and an insecticide at the same time.
5. Do not use on puppies under three months of age, nursing mothers, or sick or debilitated dogs.
6. If it appears that a dog has been accidentally overdosed, take it and the insecticide container immediately to the nearest veterinary hospital. If a veterinarian cannot be reached quickly, bathe the animal and remove all traces of the insecticide.

FLEA CONTROL MEDICATIONS

Fleas and other external parasites can be controlled by the use of oral medications which are available in tablet and liquid form. These are prescription drugs and can be obtained only through a veterinarian. They are organophosphate systemic insecticides, which are rapidly absorbed and distributed throughout the dog's tissues. Fleas and other biting insects are killed when they ingest the drug upon biting the dog. While the manufacturers claim the first week of treatment kills 95% of the fleas, and that additional weeks of treatment will remove all the fleas from the dog, the fact is that success with these products depends on using them before the flea population becomes too large.

One such product is Proban, manufactured by Haver-Lockhart Laboratories. Another is Ectoral, manufactured by Pitman-Moore Company. Depending on which drug is used, the dosage is given either twice a week, or every other day. Used in special instances—under veterinary supervision, in the smallest possible dosage for a limited period of time, and in healthy dogs that can tolerate them—they have not been found to be harmful. They are effective, if used early in the flea season, when the flea population is still small.

Although these drugs sound like the ideal solution for flea control, they are not without hazard to the dog. No other insecticides, pesticides, or similar-acting drugs should be used on dogs receiving these products or overdosage may occur. Nor should flea medications be used in greyhounds (they are overly sensitive to them), in pregnant, nursing, young, or sick dogs, or in dogs under stress or having surgery. Atropine is the antidote if signs of overdosage (vomiting, muscle tremors, salivation, and diarrhea) are seen.

Use of systemic insecticides seems a reasonable approach to flea control, but many veterinarians and dog owners have been reluctant to use them because of possible toxic side effects. However, no serious toxicity or side effects have been reported in clinical trials or by veterinary practitioners using these products, and the margin of safety for them is high.

PUBLIC HEALTH AND CANINE PARASITES

Because of generally high standards of hygiene, the incidence of human infections from dog roundworms and tapeworms is small today. However, there are some dangers, particularly to children, from the canine internal parasites. The following are the most frequently encountered:

ROUNDWORMS If a child ingests a roundworm egg, a condition called *visceral larva migrans* (which, freely translated, means "larva in migration through the viscera," or internal organs) can occur. The larvae of dog roundworms do not grow to adult worms in humans. However, when these larvae from roundworm eggs are released in the human intestine, they enter the intestinal wall and from there migrate through other tissues and organs of the body. During this migration, the larvae can cause damage, particularly to the liver, lungs, nervous system, and eyes. While there are usually no dramatic symptoms, fever, poor appetite, muscle pains, coughing, and irritability have been reported. Although almost all children recover without treatment, cases that involve the eye may be serious, as they can lead to impaired vision.

TAPEWORMS   People can become infected with the flea tapeworm if they swallow an infected dog flea. While this is uncommon, cases have been reported in children. Segments of the worm will be passed in the stool (*see* Tapeworms, earlier in this chapter, for description). Treatment with medication will be required to eliminate the worms in such instances.

The larvae of some dog tapeworms can encyst (become enclosed in a sac) in humans and cause tissue damage or allergic reactions.

HOOKWORMS   Dog hookworms do not infect humans, but the larvae can penetrate human skin and set up a local skin irritation, called *cutaneous larva migrans,* or more descriptively "creeping eruptions." Local treatment is effective.

HEARTWORMS   There have been rare reports of heartworms infecting humans; however, the worms do not usually mature, but become encysted in the lungs.

PINWORMS   Despite the fact that many people—and even some MDs—believe that pinworms come from dogs or cats, this worm infects only humans and some primates.

3

Allergies

Allergies in dogs are similar to allergies in humans. They can manifest themselves in a variety of ways, depending on which area of the body reacts, in nose and eye discharges, sneezing, digestive upsets, and skin lesions (sores). Most cases of skin disease in dogs are caused by one allergy or another. Compared to its occurrence in humans, allergic asthma is uncommon, but it is similar in symptoms when it does occur.

Veterinary clients frequently question a diagnosis of allergy in an adult dog that has not previously had any problems, but it must be emphasized that dogs, like people, can develop allergies at any age and the signs can appear quite suddenly.

ALLERGIES IN DOGS

An allergy is a hypersensitive reaction to allergy-causing substances known as allergens or antigens. In sensitive individuals the body produces antibodies when first exposed to an allergen, but there are no allergic symptoms. On subsequent exposure, the antigen and antibody interact, and this results in symptoms. Normally antibodies produced by the body, are—in vaccinations, for example—protective, but in allergic individuals the immune mechanism malfunctions and also overreacts.

The most common causes of allergy in dogs are:

- *Pollens and molds,* which cause hay fever or seasonal-type allergies.
- *Flea saliva.* While dogs not allergic to fleas can have hundreds of fleas and hardly scratch at all, the presence of only a few fleas on allergic dogs causes intense itching. The reaction may occur only seasonally in climate zones where fleas are eliminated by the cold, or in the excessive dryness of desert heat.
- *Chemicals,* such as those found in soaps, waxes, carpets, and flea collars. This type of hypersensitivity is known as contact allergy.
- *Insect bites and stings.*
- *Foods.* German shepherds, in particular, may be affected.

Symptoms

Itching is the main sign of allergic skin disease in a dog. The affected skin is red and moist in patches; these areas are often referred to as "hot spots." In the early stages, flea allergies are most evident over the back and tail.

Allergies to pollen and molds usually cause some eye and nose discharge, and skin lesions are often present on the face and front legs. The dog will often lick its paws and rub its face with its paws. The saliva keeps these areas chronically moist, and in time the hairs on light-colored dogs will turn rust-colored or pinkish from the saliva and the moisture.

Contact allergies are seen where the dog's coat is thin or nonexistent: the armpits, chin, elbows, hocks, foot pads, abdomen, and genitals. Dogs allergic to flea collars will show irritation around the neck.

Food allergies cause diarrhea and sometimes also skin lesions.

Diagnosis

The dog's case history is often diagnostic in itself, particularly if the condition is seasonal. In skin allergies the intense itching and the location of the lesions are helpful in diagnosis.

Elimination diets are used to diagnose food allergies.

In all allergies, response to treatment is often used as a guide to diagnosis.

Intradermal skin testing, which involves injection of a suspected allergen, is now conducted by many veterinarians to determine what specifically is causing the dog's allergic symptoms. Patch and scratch testing are similar to intradermal testing except that the antigen is applied to the skin. Skin testing is not essential in all cases, nor is it 100% reliable, and it is seldom of value in testing for food allergies.

Treatment

For allergies there are three basic methods of treatment:

Avoidance of the cause. While not always practical as a method of allergy treatment, avoidance is most effective when it can be applied.

Treatment of symptoms. This may involve the use of corticosteroid drugs by the veterinarian to relieve the symptoms. In skin allergies these drugs relieve the intense itching, and this stops the self-mutilation. The dog owner will then have to give the drugs in tablet form, in decreasing dosages, usually for a few months. It is important that the dog be maintained on the smallest possible dosage that relieves the symptoms, as these are very potent drugs with undesirable side effects when not used according to directions. (*See* Chapter 17, Drugs; Corticosteroids.)

In flea allergy, the fleas on the dog and in its environment need to be controlled by means of insecticides. (*See* Chapter 2, Parasites; External Parasites: Fleas, Flea Control.)

Antihistamines and tranquilizers are also used to treat allergies in dogs, but they are not nearly as effective in relieving allergic symptoms in dogs as they are in people.

Contact allergies require the removal of the allergy-causing substance by shampooing.

Food allergies are similarly controlled by identifying the

cause through an elimination diet, and then removing the offending food(s) from the diet.

Desensitization (hyposensitization). This is another approach to allergy control. Once a correct diagnosis by skin testing has been made, then increasingly large doses of the allergy-causing substance are given to the dog by injection at varying intervals for up to five months. The dog's body builds up antibodies to counteract the substance to which he is allergic. Unfortunately, this is not a quick process, nor is it always effective.

Allergic skin diseases that do not respond to conventional treatments or are very advanced when first seen by the veterinarian may be treated by injections of refined cobra venom, surgery, radiation, or injections of corticosteroids directly into the lesions.

ALLERGIC SKIN DISEASES (*See* Chapter 4, The Skin; Allergic Skin Diseases.)

FOOD ALLERGIES

If a dog is vomiting and producing a stool that is soft to watery in consistency, particularly when certain foods are fed, a food allergy can be suspected. Other causes of these symptoms must, of course, be ruled out. Skin lesions may also occur with food allergies.

Diagnosis and Treatment

To diagnose a food allergy, the dog is placed on a hypoallergenic diet consisting of foods either not commonly fed to the dog or known to have a low probability of causing an allergy. The dog will be kept on this diet for five days, at which time a new selected food will be added to the diet for five days. If an allergic response occurs, the new food is removed and the dog is put back on the hypoallergenic diet for five more days, or until allergy symptoms subside. This testing of new foods every five days is continued until enough nonallergenic foods are identified to permit a veterinarian to design a nonallergenic diet for the dog.

A commercially produced hypoallergenic diet, Prescription Diet, d/d made by Hill's, is available through your veterinarian, or the dog owner can use a homemade diet such as:

4 ounces cooked lamb (no seasoning, discard excess fat)	1½ teaspoons dicalcium phosphate
1 cup cooked rice	Vitamin and mineral supplements to meet daily requirements
1 teaspoon corn oil	

This formula produces three-quarters of a pound of food. Feed enough to maintain normal body weight: a five-pound dog would require approximately one-third pound per day; a twenty-pound dog, one pound; a forty-pound dog, one and a half pounds; and a hundred-pound dog, three pounds.

Sometimes even the most carefully controlled elimination diet testing fails to identify the allergy-causing foods, and in these instances corticosteroids may be necessary to control the symptoms.

HIVES

Hives, *urticaria,* appear on the skin as slightly raised patches or wheals which are redder or paler than the surrounding skin. In dogs hives usually cause itching and are seen most frequently on the head and face. The most common causes in dogs are vaccination reactions, food allergies, or penicillin allergies.

TREATMENT Most cases of hives are not serious, and the skin swellings usually disappear within twenty-four hours. The cause, if known, should be eliminated. Antihistamines are effective in mild cases. If the skin reaction is severe and worsens, then an injection of epinephrine by your veterinarian will be necessary. Corticosteroids are sometimes used to prevent relapses.

ANAPHYLAXIS

Anaphylaxis is an exaggerated allergic reaction, often referred to as anaphylactic shock. In sensitive individuals it can be induced by many different agents, such as drugs, vaccines, insect bites, and foods. Fortunately, anaphylaxis is relatively rare in dogs.

SYMPTOMS The signs of anaphylactic shock develop immediately or within a few minutes of exposure. The symptoms are trembling, vomiting, diarrhea, shortness of breath; sometimes the skin will redden and hives will occur. The dog will collapse in shock and die in less than thirty minutes.

TREATMENT Emergency treatment is essential in anaphylactic shock. Epinephrine and antihistamine injections may reverse the symptoms if given at once. Treatment for shock, including the use of oxygen and blood transfusions, will also be required. Often dogs cannot be saved, as death occurs so quickly.

4

The Skin

DEALING WITH SKIN DISEASES IN DOGS

Excluding routine physical examinations, vaccinations, and elective surgeries, the largest number of consultations in the average veterinary practice deals with skin diseases in the dog. Although seldom fatal, skin diseases are the most frustrating medical problem for veterinarians and dog owners to deal with. The causes are multiple, the signs and symptoms of many are similar, the diagnosis is often difficult, and response to any treatment can be slow or hard to evaluate. Some diseases can be controlled but not cured, and many diseases are chronic, tending to recur seasonally or when treatment is stopped.

When dealing with skin disease in a dog, good communication between the veterinarian and the dog owner is very important. The dog owner needs to understand fully the nature of the disease and the methods of treatment recommended. Frequently a breakdown in communication sends dog owners shopping from one veterinarian to another trying to find a cure for an incurable skin disease! A veterinarian may give the dog a corticosteroid injection, for example, in an allergic skin disease, and the condition will clear up completely in a few days. The owner's joy may become frustration with the veterinarian, however, when the condition recurs in a few weeks if the owner was not told to expect this. What the dog owner also needs to know is that corticosteroids are potent drugs, with many undesirable side effects, and they should not be used carelessly to treat skin diseases in dogs.

Although more costly initially, a full diagnostic work-up to identify the cause of skin disease and a detailed explanation of treatment approaches and prognosis are the best approach. The cost of continuing treatments and consultations following this should not be prohibitive, and an informed client may keep even chronic skin conditions under control with home treatment and minimal continuing veterinary expense.

Following is a discussion of the diagnostic and treatment approaches to skin disease in general and a description of the most frequently encountered skin diseases in dogs.

SKIN DISEASE DIAGNOSTIC METHODS

It is not difficult for the experienced veterinarian to make an educated guess at the diagnosis of a skin disease in a dog from a physical examination. In many cases, this is an acceptable practice; if the diagnosis is correct, the dog owner has been saved the expense of further diagnostic tests. However, if the diagnosis is incorrect, this hit-or-miss approach can be costly to the dog owner, damaging to the dog, and embarrassing to the veterinarian. With skin diseases, a confirmed diagnosis is essential for satisfactory treatment and control. The following approaches are used to diagnose skin disease in dogs:

History. The veterinarian needs a complete medical history of a dog suffering from skin disease, and the dog owner can be most helpful in this area by answering all questions. Beyond the dog's age, sex, and breed, a dog owner may be asked the following:

- What is the dog's previous medical history?
- When did the skin condition start?
- Is the condition seasonal?

- Are people or other pets in the household affected?
- Has the dog been exposed to insecticides, grasses, new bedding, chemicals, a new environment, etc.?
- Where did the skin lesions start? Are they spreading?
- Is there itching, licking, and scratching?
- What is the dog being fed? Has there been a change in diet lately?
- Are the appetite and bowel functions normal?
- Does your dog have any internal or external parasites?
- Is the dog's behavior normal? Is it more active or more depressed than usual?

Physical examination. The veterinarian will give the dog a general physical examination, with specific attention to the location, distribution, and type of skin lesions; hair condition and loss; parasites or signs of parasites; and evidence of self-inflicted trauma.

Skin scrapings. If the veterinarian suspects microscopic skin parasites, such as mange mites, or an infection such as ringworm, a skin scraping is called for. The test involves taking a superficial scraping of the skin from the dog and examining it under the microscope. The test is not very painful, and most dogs are cooperative patients for this procedure. A number of scrapings may be required to reach a diagnosis.

Wood's light examination. Since the affected hairs of dogs infected with some species of ringworm fungal organisms give off a yellow-green fluorescence, the veterinarian may order a Wood's light examination, which requires a special ultraviolet light used in a dark room.

Bacterial and fungal cultures. If the veterinarian suspects the skin disease is caused by a bacterial or fungal agent, he or she will suggest a culture and sensitivity test. As in humans, culturing involves collecting bacteria or fungi with a swab, then growing the organism in the laboratory; sensitivity testing is done by adding various antibiotic-impregnated disks to the culture in order to determine which antibiotic will be most effective in treatment. Additional tests may be done to identify the specific organism causing the disease, as this can be useful in the choice of treatment.

Skin biopsy. Biopsy involves the removal of skin tissues and the examination of them, usually microscopically, in order to establish a precise diagnosis. While used most commonly to identify skin tumors, it can be helpful in diagnosing difficult skin disease cases as well.

Blood tests. Blood tests can be helpful in diagnosing some skin diseases, particularly those of allergic or parasitic origin. Certain white blood cells called eosinophils increase in numbers in parasitic and allergic skin diseases. Blood tests are also indicated in some bacterial skin diseases or in those which affect the dog's general health.

Allergy testing. Many veterinarians now use skin tests to determine if the dog is allergic. Small amounts of the most common allergy-causing substances (antigens) are injected or scratched into the skin. If the area of injection swells and reddens, the reaction is positive, and the dog is most likely allergic to the substance. Although this testing is not 100% reliable diagnostically—false positives and cross-reactions may occur—it is most helpful if other diagnostic measures have not been informative, or if response to treatment has been poor.

Response to treatment. If the dog owner either does not want or cannot afford to spend much money on diagnostic tests, an experienced veterinarian can often make a diagnosis on the basis of response to treatment.

SKIN DISEASE TREATMENTS

Successful treatment of skin disease in dogs depends on accurate diagnosis. Current treatments for skin diseases in dogs include:

Topical treatments. The first approach, particularly if the skin disease is localized, is to clip the hair away from the affected area. Following this, a medicated shampoo is usually recommended to remove scabs, crusts, dirt, skin scales, discharges, and other debris. Medicated lotions, powders, creams, or ointments may be applied to the lesions, although not all skin diseases require or are aided by such local treatment. These medications may contain drying agents, skin softeners, soothing agents, keratolytic agents (which soften, dissolve, and lead to the peeling of the thickened layer of skin), antibiotics, antifungal agents, antiparasitic agents, and corticosteroids.

Overtreatment is more often a problem than undertreatment in skin diseases and can interfere with the natural healing processes. Generally, skin lesions should not be bandaged, as this retards healing; however, if severe self-inflicted trauma is occurring and no other means of control is effective, bandaging may be preferred.

Antibiotics. Many antibiotics are used in treating skin diseases, particularly those caused by bacterial infections or complicated by secondary bacterial infections. The antibiotics may be given by injection or orally, and they are often included in topical preparations.

Antifungal agents. For ringworm, griseofulvin is the drug of choice; it is administered by mouth. Treatment may be prolonged, in some cases up to six months. Tolnaftate and neomycin are used in topical treatment.

Corticosteroids. The many different corticosteroid drugs are very effective in treating skin diseases because of their anti-inflammatory and antipruritic (ease itching) effects. However, while they give dramatic relief to the itching, scratching dogs, and they impress the dog owner, they are not curative. They are potent drugs, and have many undesirable side effects; they have also been overused and abused in the treatment of canine skin diseases. Corticosteroids are essential in treating many skin diseases in dogs, but they should be used at the lowest effective dosage over the shortest period of time.

In a few chronic skin diseases, long-term use is unavoidable. The drugs must not be stopped abruptly; dogs taking them must be weaned from them gradually by giving reduced dosages over four to six weeks. (For information on safe usage *see* Chapter 17, Drugs, Corticosteroids.)

Hormones. Hormone drugs may be used to treat skin diseases that result from deficiencies or imbalances of the naturally produced hormones of the body, such as those of the thyroid, the testicles (testosterone), the ovaries (estrogen), and the adrenal and pituitary glands (adrenocortical hormones).

Prevention of self-inflicted trauma. Sedatives, tranquilizers, analgesics, and anti-itching agents are all used to prevent self-mutilation in skin diseases in dogs. Also used are safe but bad-tasting topical preparations, and mechanical devices, such as Elizabethan collars, which prevent the dog from licking the body or scratching the ears and face. Although antihistamines are not very effective in relieving skin disease symptoms in dogs, they are sometimes used for their sedative effects.

Insecticides. Insecticidal powders, sprays, dips, shampoos, liquids, and ointments are used to treat parasitic skin diseases in dogs. Fumigation and spraying will also be needed to remove external parasites from the dog's environment. (*See also* Chapter 2, Parasites; External Parasites: Fleas, Flea Control.)

Nutrition. Good nutrition is important in treating all diseases. Some skin diseases are caused by food allergies and in these cases, the offending food should be eliminated from the diet. Dry, scaly skin and dry hair can be due to a lack of polyunsaturated fatty acids in the diet. The B-vitamins and vitamins A and E are also important in maintaining a healthy skin.

Surgery. Surgical intervention is occasionally required in skin diseases to repair severe lesions, usually caused by self-inflicted trauma, and to drain abscesses. Skin tumors, particularly if malignant, must be removed surgically.

Hyposensitization. Also called desensitization, this is being used with increasing frequency in veterinary practice for treating allergic skin diseases. (*See also* Chapter 3, Allergies; Desensitization.) This is not a quick process, nor is it always effective, but some good results have been obtained. It has the added advantage that the dog will not have to be kept on corticosteroid drugs. There are some hazards associated with this procedure, so careful observation for adverse reactions is important following each injection.

ALLERGIC SKIN DISEASES

Atopic Dermatitis (Hay Fever)

Atopy is an allergic disease to which a dog may have a hereditary predisposition. It is caused by allergens in the environment, which enter the body through the respiratory and gastrointestinal tracts. Most of these diseases are seasonal and approximate hay fever allergies in humans.

Grass and weed allergens appear to be the main cause of these allergies in dogs. The history is diagnostic: The dog gets the symptoms at the same time each year and is not bothered during the winter months. The disease may become chronic, and then it can be continuous and no longer seasonal. Dust and mold allergies are also continuous. Dalmatians, poodles, terriers, and dachshunds are the breeds most often affected.

SYMPTOMS The symptoms include some sneezing and eye discharges, but the major symptoms are face rubbing, foot licking, and scratching the armpits. Most of the skin lesions are the result of self-mutilation from rubbing and scratching.

DIAGNOSIS Diagnosis is based on the history and is confirmed by skin allergy testing.

TREATMENT Treatment involves avoidance of the allergens, use of corticosteroids, and hyposensitization. The disease can be controlled with treatment, but there is no cure.

Flea Allergy Dermatitis

Flea allergy dermatitis (FAD) is the major cause of skin disease in dogs in areas of moderate temperatures below 5,000 feet elevation. Many dog owners refer to this as "the summer itch." The cause is a hypersensitivity or allergy to flea saliva.

SYMPTOMS The major symptom is intense itching. In susceptible dogs the presence of even one flea can cause great discomfort. The skin lesions show up first over the top of the tail, where it joins the back, and spread towards the head along the back. The area becomes reddened first, and then pustules and crusts form. There may be some hair loss. There is intense itching, and the dog continually licks and tears at the affected areas, or rubs his back against furniture and rolls on his back. If the condition becomes chronic, the skin thickens and darkens in color.

DIAGNOSIS Diagnosis is based on the history, clinical signs, response to eliminating fleas on the dog and in the dog's environment, and skin allergy testing.

TREATMENT Treatment is, in theory, very simple: Eradicate fleas. However, this is by no means an easy task (*see* Chapter 2, Parasites; External Parasites: Fleas, Flea Control). Medicated shampoos, corticosteroids, and topical medications may also be required to control the disease. Hyposensitization may also be used in treatment, as some good responses have been reported.

Contact Dermatitis

Contact dermatitis, as the name suggests, is a skin disease caused by an allergic reaction to an agent the dog has contacted, such as shampoos, insecticides, carpets, floor waxes, petroleum products, dyes, poison oak or ivy, and plastics.

SYMPTOMS The signs are itching and the appearance of skin lesions in the areas of contact, most often the feet, chin, legs, lower abdomen, and genital areas. Hairless areas are more susceptible.

DIAGNOSIS The diagnosis is based on the fast onset and the location of the lesions. Allergy skin testing can be used, but is not always practical; investigative work by the owner often pinpoints the offending agent.

TREATMENT Treatment involves the removal of the cause, a bath to remove the agent from the dog's skin and haircoat, and the use of corticosteroids, orally or in topical form, if the skin reaction is severe and the dog is mutilating the affected areas.

Food Allergy

Sometimes food allergy also causes skin lesions. (*See* Chapter 3, Allergies; Food Allergies).

BACTERIAL SKIN DISEASES (PYODERMAS)

Skin diseases caused by bacteria are usually recognized by the presence of pus discharges and are called pyodermas. The bacteria most often causing pyodermas are the staphylococcus and streptococcus organisms.

Impetigo

SYMPTOMS Impetigo is a superficial bacterial skin infection characterized by pinhead-sized pustules, most evident in the hairless areas of the dog. It is a disease of young dogs. The affected areas do not itch, and unlike the disease in humans, canine impetigo is not contagious to other dogs or people.

TREATMENT Medicated baths, topical ointments, attention to nutrition, and elimination of internal parasites will resolve most cases.

Acne

SYMPTOMS Acne in dogs is similar to the same condition in humans. It is seen most often in young dogs and usually clears up when they reach sexual maturity. The chin, neck, and lower lips are involved, and redness, swelling, and black-heads are evident. Pustules form if naturally occurring bacteria on the skin infect the acne lesions.

TREATMENT   Treatment in severe cases includes clipping the hair in the affected areas, gentle scrubbing with antiseptic soaps, antibiotic ointments, and oral antibiotics. Vitamin A-related chemicals, both topically and orally, are now being used with success in human cases of acne.

Pyodermas

SYMPTOMS   Pyodermas are pus-discharging skin diseases. Early in the disease the skin is reddened, but as the disease progresses, the area becomes ulcerated, pustules develop and discharge pus, scabs and crusts form, and hair loss is usual. The lesions may be superficial or deep, and sometimes the infection spreads throughout the body leading to a generalized illness. In obese dogs and dogs of the pug-nosed breeds, pyodermas are frequently seen in the skin fold areas of the face, lips, and vulva. Other areas affected in dogs are the nose and between the toes, and in heavier breeds of dogs, the elbows and hocks. A pyoderma of the abdominal area is often seen in young puppies.

DIAGNOSIS   Diagnosis is made by the history, and the appearance and location of the lesions. Bacterial culture and sensitivity testing may be recommended to determine which antibiotics will be effective in treatment. In generalized disease, blood tests will be required. Occasionally a skin biopsy is called for to confirm the diagnosis in difficult cases.

TREATMENT   Treatment involves clipping the hair in the affected areas, cleaning the lesions with antiseptic soaps, antibiotic ointments, and using injectable or oral antibiotics. Cases with extensive lesions will need medicated baths. Corticosteroids are required in some cases if itching is present and cannot be alleviated by other methods; the drugs must be used with care, however, if generalized infection is present. Occasionally surgery is required in pyodermas involving deep skin folds. Custom-made vaccines have been tried in long-standing cases with some reported success. Most cases respond to treatment, but recurrences are not uncommon, so follow-up home and preventive treatments may be required on a long-term basis.

Skin Abscess

A skin abscess is a localized condition of pus under the skin, and is not technically a skin disease. Abscesses in dogs, unlike cats, are relatively rare. They are caused by bacteria being carried into a wound, most commonly from a bite or a foreign body such as a plant awn.

SYMPTOMS The area becomes hot, painful, and swollen, and in most cases will eventually open and discharge pus.

TREATMENT Many abscesses will heal without treatment if the dog owner makes sure the abscess is fully drained and keeps the area clean with local washing and antiseptics. Moist hot compresses can be used in the early stages to bring the abscess to a head.

Abscesses require veterinary medical and/or surgical treatment if they are causing generalized illness, contain a foreign body, or are spreading under the skin into a condition called cellulitis. Surgical drainage, removal of dead and infected tissues, and antibiotics will then be required.

PARASITIC SKIN DISEASES

Sarcoptic Mange (Canine Scabies)

Sarcoptic mange is a skin disease of dogs caused by a microscopic eight-legged mite called *Sarcoptes scabiei* var. *canis*. The mite spends its entire life on the dog and only survives a few days if separated from it. The female burrows into the skin and lays a few eggs daily. The eggs hatch in one week as larvae, develop into nymphs, and then become adults in a few weeks.

SYMPTOMS   This disease causes the most severe itching of all skin diseases in dogs. Initially there is loss of hair and some reddening of the affected areas, and later raised bumps and crusting of the skin are evident. The lesions are seen most frequently on the edges of the ears, the elbows, the head, the lower chest, and the abdomen. Most of the skin damage is a result of self-mutilation due to the intense itching.

DIAGNOSIS   Diagnosis is made from the history, clinical signs, location of the lesions, and the intense itching, and is confirmed by microscopically identifying the mites in a skin scraping.

TREATMENT   Treatment involves the use of insecticidal dips weekly for up to six weeks. Medicated shampoos are used to remove the scales and crusts and prevent further skin damage. Corticosteroids by mouth and in topical medications are used to relieve the intense itching. Most cases respond favorably if the treatment is continued for a long enough period of time.

CONTAGION   Canine scabies is highly contagious, so other dogs in the household should be checked. Although the mite is species-specific and only causes disease in dogs, it can be

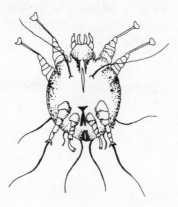

Sarcoptic Mange Mite
(Enlarged)

transferred to humans. In people the mite can burrow into the skin and cause red bumps which persist for up to three weeks, but it does not reproduce, so there is no further spread of the disease. Many dog owners with these lesions will ask the veterinarian to treat them as well as the dog, but veterinarians are not licensed to treat humans. However, your veterinarian can give you a note for your physician, stating that your skin lesions look suspiciously like canine scabies.

Demodectic Mange (Red Mange)

Demodectic mange is caused by a microscopic carrot-shaped mite called *Demodex canis*. The mite lives in the hair follicles. Most dogs have some demodectic mites, but they only cause disease in dogs with depressed immune systems. The young are most often affected.

SYMPTOMS The skin disease is usually mild, and localized hair loss, with slight reddening and scaling of the skin, are the only obvious signs. There is no itching, which helps to distinguish it from scabies. The front legs and the face, especially around the eyes, are most often affected. A few cases become generalized, with secondary bacterial infections complicating the disease, and this can result in a serious illness.

DIAGNOSIS The diagnosis is made by the appearance and location of the lesions, and is confirmed by a skin scraping and in some cases by biopsy. Culture and sensitivity testing may be required if the disease is complicated by a pyoderma.

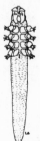

Demodectic Mange Mite (Enlarged)

TREATMENT   Treatment involves the use of insecticidal ointments on the lesions. In generalized disease, clipping, insecticidal dips, shampooing, ointments, and oral and topical antibiotics will be required. Some cases respond well to oral systemic insecticides. (*See* Chapter 2, Parasites; External Parasites: Flea Control Medications.) Corticosteroids are not recommended in cases of demodectic mange because most affected dogs are already immuno-depressed—nor are they often required, unless self-mutilation is occurring. The response to treatment in demodectic mange is generally good and many dogs recover without treatment. The generalized disease has a poorer prognosis and some dogs just cannot be cured and may have to be euthanized after months of treatment.

CONTAGION   Demodectic mange is not considered contagious to other dogs or to humans, although newborn pups can be infected from the mother. The majority of dogs harbor some of these mites without showing any signs of disease.

Cheyletiella Dermatitis

The *Cheyletiella* species of mites do not burrow, but live on the surface of the skin, and can infect dogs, cats, and humans.

SYMPTOMS   These mites do not cause itching as intense as sarcoptic mange mites, and mostly affect puppies, leading to a scaly, dandruff-like condition.

DIAGNOSIS   The diagnosis is made by the symptoms, and confirmed by a skin scraping.

TREATMENT   Treatment is the same as that for sarcoptic mange. Most cases clear up quickly with treatment.

CONTAGION   People are only infected by very close and prolonged contact with an infected dog.

Ear Mites (See Chapter 6, The Ears; Ear Mites.)

**Skin Diseases Caused by Lice, Ticks, Fleas, and Flies
(See Chapter 2, Parasites: External Parasites.)**

FUNGAL SKIN DISEASES

There are a number of fungi that cause skin disease in dogs, but only ringworm will be discussed here because it causes 99% of fungal skin problems in dogs, and the other fungal diseases affect other areas of the body as well as the skin.

Ringworm

The fungi which cause ringworm in dogs are microscopic, algae-like organisms that produce spores. The species which infect dogs are *Microsporum canis, Microsporum gypseum,* and *Trichophyton mentagrophytes.*

SYMPTOMS   Ringworm is seen mostly in young dogs and causes loss of hair, usually in circular patches; hence the name "ringworm," although it actually has nothing to do with a worm! The fungi invade only the dead tissue of the skin, hair, and nails. The center of the circular skin patches may show crusting, and also pus if there is bacterial infection present. Early lesions are seen most often on the head and limbs, but the disease can spread over the rest of the body and into the nails. There is little itching, so self-mutilation is seldom a problem.

DIAGNOSIS   Diagnosis is made by the history and the appearance of the lesions, and is confirmed by a Wood's light test, a skin scraping, and culturing the fungi. *Microsporum canis* fluoresces under the Wood's lamp, but only about 50% of such cases show up as positive to this test, and since some drugs and chemicals can cause hair to fluoresce and lead to false positives, this test is not used alone to make a diagnosis.

TREATMENT   Treatment is with a drug called griseofulvin, which is very effective, but may need to be administered for months to cure the disease. It is given by mouth, either daily, or in massive doses every week to ten days. Other treatments involve clipping the hair around the lesions, the use of medicated shampoos, and antifungal ointments. The response to treatment is good in most cases.

CONTAGION   Ringworm is contagious to other dogs, to cats, and to humans, particularly children. Other pets in the household should be checked and treated if infected. Sometimes other pets are given a single dose of griseofulvin as a preventive. Affected pets should, of course, be handled carefully by adults, and isolated from other pets and children until no longer infective.

Infection in people is seldom severe; a few reddened ring-shaped skin lesions may be seen on the arms or legs. Local treatment with over-the-counter antifungal agents, such as tolnaftate (Tinactin) will clear up most cases, but if the lesions spread, a visit to your physician will be necessary.

HORMONAL SKIN DISEASES

The effects of hormones on skin can be complex and difficult to diagnose. The thyroid gland, pituitary gland, adrenal glands, testicles, and ovaries all produce hormones which if excessive (hyper), deficient (hypo), or out of balance produce changes in the skin and haircoat. The characteristics of all hormonal skin problems are: loss of hair in an evenly distributed pattern on each side of the body, darkening of the skin, no pruritus (itching), and a chronic duration. The skin changes are just one symptom of hormonal abnormalities; other body systems are also affected and the signs related to these may be more diagnostic than the skin changes.

Hypothyroidism

The thyroid gland produces thyroid hormone, which regulates cell metabolism. In hypothyroidism, there is a deficiency of this hormone, caused by reduction in size or destruction of the gland. The exact reason this occurs is not always evident or understood. Hypothyroidism is seen most frequently in four- to six-year-old, medium to large breeds of dogs; miniature and toy breeds are seldom affected.

SYMPTOMS The signs of hypothyroidism are lethargy, increased appetite, weight gain, loss of libido, infertility, sensitivity to cold, a brittle, dry, dull haircoat, loss of hair especially over the neck, back, and tail areas, and in some cases an oily skin and excessive wax in the ears. As the disease advances, the skin darkens in color, thickens, and feels cool to the touch; the dog becomes more dull and irritable, and heart problems may develop. Only about 50% of hypothyroid dogs show the skin and haircoat changes.

DIAGNOSIS Diagnosis is made by laboratory blood tests that measure the thyroid hormone levels.

TREATMENT Treatment involves the use of replacement thyroid hormone drugs, usually for life. Establishing the dosage requires veterinary supervision, and periodic monitoring of an affected dog is necessary. If the diagnosis is correct, the prognosis is good.

Hyperadrenocorticism

This disease is also called Cushing's syndrome, named after the man who first recognized the problem. There are a number of different adrenal hormones, all of which regulate metabolism. In hyperadrenocorticism, there is excessive secretion of these hormones due to disease of the adrenal glands themselves or to malfunction of the pituitary gland, which controls the adrenal glands. The cause is not always understood, but tumors of either of these glands can result in hyperadrenocorticism. Excessive use of corticosteroid drugs over long periods of time is the most frequently recognized cause in veterinary medicine.

SYMPTOMS   Signs of this disorder include symmetrical hair loss over the body (although the face and legs are not affected except in advanced cases), darkening of the skin, a pendulous abdomen even though the dog is thin, excessive thirst and urination, and increased appetite. Later signs include lethargy, weakness, bone pain, poor wound healing, easy bruising, and liver problems. Calcium deposits may also occur in the skin and this is a very diagnostic sign of this disease.

DIAGNOSIS   Diagnosis is made by blood tests, which show changes in the white blood cell counts, high glucose levels, and high serum cholesterol. More expensive blood and urine tests to measure the hormone levels can be done to confirm the diagnosis.

TREATMENT   Treatment involves the use of drugs to reduce the hormone output of the adrenal glands. Removal of the glands surgically is another approach to treatment, and is essential if the cause is from tumors of the glands. Replacement hormones will then need to be given for the life of the dog. The prognosis is not very good, but some dogs do well with treatment. Most will die if not treated.

Male Dogs—Sex Hormone Problems

The most frequently encountered skin problem in male dogs related to sex hormones is the overproduction of estrogen (female hormone), which causes feminization of the dog. One cause is a tumor of the testicles, called a Sertoli cell tumor; in other cases the testicles appear normal and the cause is unknown.

SYMPTOMS   Signs include a loss of hair, particularly on the flanks and in the genital area, mammary gland enlargement and sometimes milk production, lack of libido, attractiveness to other male dogs, darkening and thickening of the skin, oiliness of the skin, and excessive wax in the ears. If the cause is from a tumor, the affected testicle will be enlarged, but often the testicle is retained in the abdomen and cannot be seen.

DIAGNOSIS   Diagnosis is made by response to treatment.

TREATMENT   Castration is recommended, particularly if a tumor is suspected. A replacement testosterone (male hormone) injection may be given. Medicated shampoos and ear cleaning will help improve the skin condition. Corticosteroids can be used as an alternative to castration if the cause is not from a tumor and, in some cases, may be required following castration.

Female Dogs—Sex Hormone Problems

Hyperestrogenism. Hyperestrogenism is the production of too much estrogen in the female dog, and is most commonly due to cysts on the ovaries.

SYMPTOMS   There is loss of hair on the flanks and genital areas, and later on the abdomen and under the elbows. The skin darkens, becomes oily, and the ears produce excessive wax. Infertility, false pregnancy, and enlargement of the vulva and the mammary glands with milk production are other common symptoms.

DIAGNOSIS   Diagnosis is made by the symptoms, since tests to measure the estrogen levels are complicated and expensive.

TREATMENT   The best treatment is an ovariohysterectomy (spay). Medicated shampoos and ear treatments are also recommended. The prognosis is good in the majority of cases and response is seen about three weeks after surgery.

Hypoestrogenism. Hypoestrogenism is a condition caused by too low production of estrogen and is seen most often in dogs which have been spayed.

SYMPTOMS   There is a gradual loss and thinning of the hair starting in the genital and lower abdominal areas, and eventually spreading to the chest, neck, and ears. The skin is soft and smooth, and the haircoat is very fine. The nipples and vulva are small, and there may be dribbling of urine.

DIAGNOSIS Diagnosis is made by the symptoms and the history.

TREATMENT Replacement synthetic female hormones usually reverse the symptoms, although they may need to be given for a number of months before a response is noted.

Acanthosis Nigricans

Acanthosis nigricans is a chronic skin disease found mainly in dachshunds. The cause is unknown.

SYMPTOMS There is loss of hair, seen first under the elbows, darkening and thickening of the skin, and later development of an oily skin. Secondary bacterial infection of the skin is not uncommon.

DIAGNOSIS Diagnosis is made by the symptoms and by biopsy of the skin.

TREATMENT There is no known cure, and treatment is entirely supportive. It includes frequent bathing with medicated shampoos, topical medications, corticosteroids, and antibiotics if secondary infection is present. Keeping one of these dogs is hard for the owner, as constant care is required and the dogs have an unpleasant appearance and often a foul body odor.

OTHER SKIN DISEASES

There are many other skin diseases and problems in dogs, but not all can be covered due to space limitations. A brief description of some less frequently encountered skin problems follows.

Seborrhea

The sebaceous glands of the skin secrete a greasy lubricating substance. Seborrhea is a chronic skin disease which results from overproduction by these glands. The cause is unknown, although this condition often accompanies other skin diseases.

SYMPTOMS The condition has two forms: the dry form in which there is a dry scaly skin, and not much oiliness; and the greasy form in which there are oily, yellowish clumps and scales seen on the skin and hairs. There is no itching unless there is secondary bacterial infection or other skin disease involved.

DIAGNOSIS Diagnosis is based on the symptoms.

TREATMENT Cure is not possible, unless the seborrhea is caused by another skin disease that can be cured. Control involves the use of frequent medicated baths, topical medications, corticosteroids, and antibiotics if secondary infection is present.

Lick Granuloma

SYMPTOMS Lick granuloma is the development of a thickened area or nodule on a dog's leg, caused by excessive licking of the area. It is thought to be related to boredom.

TREATMENT The aim of treatment is to prevent the dog from licking the area and involves the use of bandaging, restraint collars which prevent the dog reaching the area, corticosteroids by mouth and sometimes injected into the lesion, tranquilizers, cobra venom injections into the lesion, radiation, surgical removal, and diverting the dog's attention from the area by giving the dog more playtime and exercise. It can be seen from the many suggested treatments that this can be a difficult lesion to clear up and, unfortunately, recurrences are not uncommon.

Nasal Solar Dermatitis ("Collie Nose")

SYMPTOMS Redness, loss of hair, and ulceration are seen on the nose in nasal solar dermatitis. It is called "collie nose" because collies or mixed breeds with collie ancestry are most often affected. The cause is unknown, but lack of pigment and hypersensitivity to sunlight are involved. Without treatment the condition can spread over the face.

TREATMENT Treatment consists of confinement indoors during the day, corticosteroids, antibiotics if infection is present, application of ink from a black marking pen to the nose to shield it from the sun, and, in severe cases, tattooing the nose with black ink for long-lasting protection. Sunscreen products do not usually offer enough protection. If neglected, this condition can develop into skin cancer.

Neurodermatitis

SYMPTOMS Neurodermatitis is a chronic skin inflammation aggravated by constant licking. It is not a common problem in dogs, and when it is seen, it usually involves the tail. The dog chews and bites the tail; There is loss of hair initially, and later, ulcers and crusting occur. Researchers suspect that this is due to irritation in this area caused by nervous system damage. It is possible that this damage results from earlier brain infections, most commonly following canine distemper. Boredom, anxiety neurosis, and anal sac disease have also been suggested as causes.

TREATMENT The treatment is the same as for lick granuloma. In some cases that cannot be controlled by any other approaches, the tail is amputated.

Callus

A callus is a round thickening of the skin which develops over bony pressure points in the dog. It is gray and hairless and is seen most on the elbows and hocks in large dogs, but can occur on the bottom of the chest and lower tail if the dogs lie on hard surfaces. Calluses can be prevented by providing soft bedding, but are harmless unless they become infected.

CARE OF SKIN AND HAIRCOAT

Dog owners often ask how often a dog should be bathed. In reality, unless they have a skin problem, dogs need not be bathed at all. This is because, unlike humans, they do not sweat through their skin. However, since we live closely with our dogs today, and allow them to live with us in the home, bathing at least once a month keeps the skin and haircoat clean and makes the dog a more pleasant house pet to have around. For the same reasons, dogs should be groomed—on a daily basis, if possible. All dogs shed hair, and a dog that develops a thick winter coat will shed excessively in the spring. Shedding is related to the photoperiod (light per day) and increases as the light increases. In house dogs, year-round shedding is usual because they are exposed to many hours of artificial light. The poodle breeds are said to shed less than other breeds.

The condition of a dog's skin and haircoat is related to nutrition. Some dry foods are low in fats and may need supplemental bacon fat or corn oil if the haircoat is dull and dry.

SKIN TUMORS (*See* Chapter 15, Cancer.)

5

The Eyes

The eye is the organ of vision, a complicated structure that has sometimes been compared to a camera. In reality, the eye is a lot more sophisticated than any camera ever made. The main structures and functions of the eye are:

Conjunctiva. A thin transparent membrane that covers the insides of the eyelids and part of the front of the eyeball or white of the eye. It serves a protective function.

Sclera. The strong, elastic outer coat of the eyeball, visible under the conjunctiva in the front of the human eye as the white of the eye. It protects the eye structure.

Cornea. The transparent tissue over the iris and pupil on the front of the eyeball, a continuation of the sclera that allows light to pass into the eye.

Iris. The circular colored structure of the eye, behind the cornea and in front of the lens; the iris serves to control the amount of light entering the eye by widening or contracting the pupil.

Pupil. The hole in the center of the iris, through which light enters the eye.

Lens. A transparent capsule behind the pupil, which changes shape to allow focusing on the retina.

Retina. The light-receiving inner coat at the back of the inside of the eye. It contains hundreds of nerve endings that transmit messages to the optic nerve.

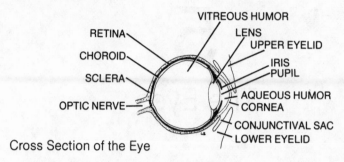

Cross Section of the Eye

Optic nerve. The nerve at the back of the eye. It conveys the messages from the retina to the seeing part of the brain, where they are then translated into the image the eye is seeing.

Aqueous humor. The clear watery fluid contained in the front chamber of the eye between the cornea and the lens. It maintains the pressure within the eye and bathes the lens.

Vitreous humor. The jelly-like fluid contained in the rear chamber of the eye between the lens and the retina. It supports the eye structures and the retina.

Choroid. The middle coat of the eye, between the retina and the sclera and continuous with the iris in front. It contains blood vessels which nourish all the eye tissues.

VETERINARY OPHTHALMOLOGY

Because of the complexity of the eye and the importance of vision for animals as well as people, the veterinary profession now has specialists, called veterinary ophthalmologists, who treat only eye disease in animals. Like their human counterparts, these are fully trained veterinarians who spend a number of years studying eye function and disease after they receive their DVM degree.

Veterinarians will soon be referring dog owners and their dogs to one of these specialists for all except very basic eye disease diagnosis and treatments, as more and more of these specialists establish practice.

Eye Examination

Any eye examination in dogs is carried out much the same way as an eye examination in humans, except that most dogs need to be tranquilized or sedated for a thorough examination. Dogs, of course, cannot tell us what they see or feel, so diagnosis of eye disease or loss of vision in dogs is made by a complete examination of the external and internal structures of the eye. The internal eye examination is conducted in a semi-darkened room, using an ophthalmoscope and other specialized instruments. It is not easy to evaluate loss of vision in dogs because they have a great ability to compensate for blindness, especially in familiar surroundings, through more extensive use of their acute senses of smell and hearing.

Vision in Dogs

A dog's normal vision is poor when compared to that of humans. Dogs have no need for close-up sight and as a result have poor focusing ability. However, dogs have a larger pupil than humans, and have superior side (peripheral) and darkness vision. A dog sees best when following a moving object; this is the type of vision that is most suited to its needs.

Studies have been done on color vision in dogs, and it has been concluded that dogs are color-blind. They see colors only as different shades of grey, in the same manner that humans perceive colors in semi-darkness.

EYE TREATMENTS

Eye disease treatments in dogs, as in humans, are by medical and surgical means.

Medical Treatments

Topical treatments. Topical eye treatment consists of applying a medicated solution or ointment to the eye. Ointments are used more often in dogs because they are easier to apply and are effective for longer periods.

To put medication into a dog's eye, steady the dog's head by placing the left hand under the muzzle. Place the left thumb at the base of the lower eyelid of the eye to be treated; then roll the lower eyelid down with the left thumb to create a cul-de-sac. With the right hand held above the eye or resting on the dog's head, place the medication (drops or ointment) into the cul-de-sac and quickly close the eyelids. Then gently massage the eyelids to distribute the medication over the eye surface. It is important not to allow the tip of the dropper or tube to touch the eye as the tip may injure the eye or become contaminated and spread an infection.

Many different topical drugs are used to treat eye disease, including cleansing solutions, artificial tears, stimulants, astringents, drugs that dilate or contract the pupil, antibiotics, corticosteroids, antihistamines, enzymes, and certain vitamins.

Oral and systemic treatments. Various drugs that affect the eye can be given orally (by mouth) or systemically (by injection).

Specialized treatments. Other specialized treatments include the application of hot and moist or cold compresses, injections into or around the eye, radiation, and bandaging.

Surgical Treatments

Extraocular surgery. This is surgery done outside the eye; such procedures involve the eyelids, conjunctiva, and cornea.

Intraocular surgery. This is surgery done inside the eyeball; such procedures involve the lens or retina.

Extraocular surgery is performed by most veterinary practitioners, but intraocular surgery is usually best done by veterinary ophthalmologists or general veterinary practitioners who have developed skill in this specialized area. If neither of these options is available, your veterinarian can arrange to perform the surgery with the assistance of an ophthalmologist from the field of human medicine.

EYELID PROBLEMS

Entropion

Entropion is an inversion or turning inward of the eyelid margins, more commonly the lower lids. It can be congenital or acquired. Congenital entropion is the most common type and is usually an inherited condition. It is seen especially in chows, bulldogs, golden and Labrador retrievers, Saint Bernards, and Irish setters. Acquired entropion is due to injury to the eyelid or to spasm of the eyelid muscles from chronic eye irritation.

SYMPTOMS When the eyelids turn inward, the eyelashes and hair injure the cornea and conjunctiva, causing pain, excessive tear production, sensitivity to light, and eventually leads to conjunctivitis and keratitis (inflammation of the cornea).

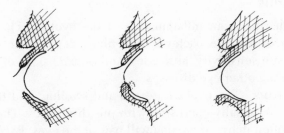

Eyelids: Normal/Entropion/Ectropion

DIAGNOSIS   Diagnosis is made by a veterinary examination of the eyelids and eyes.

TREATMENT   Congenital entropion can be corrected surgically. Acquired entropion usually corrects itself if the condition causing it is treated, although some cases may require surgical intervention as well as medical treatment.

Ectropion

Ectropion is an eversion, or turning outward, of the lower eyelid margin. It can be congenital or acquired. Congenital ectropion may be an inherited condition and is commonly seen in basset hounds, bloodhounds, cocker spaniels, and Saint Bernards. Acquired ectropion is caused by injury to the eyelid, but can also be due to damage to the facial nerve.

SYMPTOMS   The drooping lower eyelid exposes the conjunctiva and cornea, which leads to injury of these tissues. There is excessive tear production and a pustular discharge which tends to collect on the inner surface of the drooping eyelid. Conjunctivitis and keratitis (inflammation of the cornea) can be complications of severe cases of ectropion.

DIAGNOSIS   Diagnosis is made by a veterinary examination of the eyelids and eyes.

TREATMENT   Congenital ectropion can be corrected surgically. Acquired ectropion may also require surgical repair if the injury or damage to the facial nerve does not respond to medical treatments.

Blepharitis

Blepharitis is an inflammation of the eyelids. The most common causes are bacterial infections, demodectic mites, trauma, sun sensitivity, abscesses, and as extensions of or accompanying other eye diseases.

SYMPTOMS   The eyelids are red and swollen, and the lid margins are usually encrusted with pus discharges. The eyelids are often itchy, so the dog will paw at the eyes. Excessive blinking and sensitivity to light are also evident. Blepharitis is nearly always accompanied by conjunctivitis.

DIAGNOSIS Diagnosis is made by the history, symptoms, and a veterinary eye examination.

TREATMENT Treatment is directed at removing the cause. Most cases are either caused by, or accompanied by, bacterial infection, so antibiotic eye ointments are used in treatment. Flushing out the eyes and removing the encrusted discharges are also important in treatment.

Other Eyelid Problems

Distichiasis. This is a double row of eyelashes, one or both of which are turned inward against the eyeball. The condition is usually congenital. Treatment is by surgical removal of the eyelashes damaging the eyes.

Trichiasis. This is ingrowing eyelashes and is usually a congenital defect. Treatment is by surgical removal.

Third-eyelid problems. The third eyelid, also called the nictitating membrane, is located at the inner corner of the eye near the nose, and under the lower eyelid. It can become inflamed and swollen, or injured, and very often then protrudes over the visible part of the eyeball. The treatment of choice, if the condition does not respond to medical treatment, is surgical removal.

EPIPHORA (OVERFLOW OF TEARS)

Tears are formed by a special tear gland (lacrimal gland) and their function is to lubricate the cornea, supply nutrients, and carry away wastes. The tears drain out through a tear duct from the eye to the nose (naso-lacrimal duct). An abnormal overflow of tears down the cheek or face is called epiphora.

Epiphora is caused by an overproduction or an inadequate removal of tears. Epiphora is a common problem in poodles;

quite frequently it is due to an inadequate removal of tears caused by blockage of the tear ducts, although often the cause is unknown. Epiphora is seen accompanying most diseases and disorders of the eye, particularly conjunctivitis and keratitis (inflammation of the cornea). In these cases it is due to overproduction of tears from eye irritation, although sometimes there is blockage of the ducts as well.

SYMPTOMS The overflow of tears down the face or cheek is readily visible in epiphora. In dogs with light-colored or white hair, especially poodles, there is a brown staining of the hair where the tears contact the face.

DIAGNOSIS Diagnosis is made by the symptoms and a veterinary eye examination. A special test, using a staining solution, can be done to determine if the tear ducts are blocked.

Unfortunately, in poodles the cause of epiphora is not always readily determined. Sometimes a low-grade infection of the nose and throat causes partial or complete blockage of the tear ducts, and this is most likely the cause if antibiotics given by mouth and applied in ointment form in the eyes helps reduce or clear up the problem. If the epiphora recurs when the antibiotics are stopped, the tonsils will need to be checked since they may be the source of the infection.

TREATMENT If the epiphora is due to other eye diseases, such as conjunctivitis and keratitis, then treatment of these diseases will usually clear up the problem. Cases caused by blockage of the tear ducts often respond to medical treatments with antibiotic eye ointment and sometimes oral antibiotics, but many require flushing the ducts under anesthesia or surgical opening of the ducts.

In some chronic cases that do not respond to other treatments, surgical removal of the third eyelid helps reduce tear production; the disadvantage of this procedure is that the tear production may then be inadequate, and this can lead to other eye problems.

CHRONIC EPIPHORA If the cause of epiphora cannot be determined or if it becomes a chronic or recurring problem, despite treatments, the dog owner must learn to live with the problem. Although the cosmetic effect of epiphora is unattractive, the dog's eyes and health are usually not affected in such cases. Daily washing and clipping of the hair in the stained area will keep the staining to a minimum.

CONJUNCTIVITIS

Conjunctivitis is an inflammation of the conjunctiva, and is the most widely encountered eye disease in dogs. The causes are numerous and include: bacterial, fungal, and viral infections; allergies; irritation from fumes or air pollution; foreign bodies or material in the eyes; injuries to the eyes; eye parasites; hanging the head out of car windows; tumors; entropion (a turning inward of the eyelids); ectropion (a turning outward of the lower eyelids); trichiasis (a growing inward of the eyelashes); distichiasis (a double row of eyelashes); insufficient tear production (dry eye); sinusitis; and other respiratory and infectious diseases.

SYMPTOMS In conjunctivitis, the conjunctiva will appear swollen and red, instead of pink. Excessive tear production or pus-like discharges are usually seen flowing down the face. Pain will be evidenced by the dog rubbing the eye or blinking excessively.

DIAGNOSIS Diagnosis is made from symptoms and a veterinary eye examination. It is not always easy to diagnose the cause of conjunctivitis, and laboratory studies of eye discharges and eye tissue scrapings may be required in some cases. A culture of the eye discharge and sensitivity testing to determine which antibiotic to use in treatment will be required in some chronic cases.

TREATMENT Most cases can be successfully treated with eye medications and will not require extensive diagnostic procedures, although the cause may never be determined. Foreign bodies and eye parasites can usually be removed using local anesthesia and restraint, but sometimes full anesthesia is required if the foreign bodies or parasites are deeply embedded, hard to locate, or the dog is difficult to handle. Tumors and eyelid problems will need surgical treatment. Artificial tears will be used to treat dry eye.

KERATITIS (INFLAMMATION OF THE CORNEA)

Keratitis is an inflammation of the cornea. The cornea—the clear transparent layer that covers the front of the eyeball—has no blood vessels in it and must remain clear for the dog to see adequately. When the cornea is damaged, it becomes cloudy, which interferes with sight. During the healing process, blood vessels grow into the cornea and further interfere with sight.

Keratitis is common in dogs with prominent eyes, which are more prone to injury. The causes of keratitis are the same as those of conjunctivitis, and the two conditions are frequently seen together.

SYMPTOMS The symptoms of keratitis depend on how deeply the inflammation penetrates the cornea. The eye is painful and the dog will paw at the eye or rub it against objects. There is usually an eye discharge which may be due to overproduction of tears from the eye irritation or may be pus-like if a bacterial infection is involved. The dog is also sensitive to light and will blink excessively. The cornea may appear cloudly as the condition advances and small pus-discharging ulcers may be visible on the cornea.

DIAGNOSIS Diagnosis is made by symptoms and a veterinary eye examination. Your veterinarian will need to determine the extent of the corneal injury and how deeply it penetrates the cornea, and will use special eye stain tests to make the lesions more visible.

TREATMENT The aim of treatment is to restore the cornea to a clear membrane. Most cases respond to medical treatment with eye ointments if the initial cause is treated or removed, but a few will require surgical cautery or repair of the corneal lesions, particularly if they are deep. The cornea will never be good as new, and for this reason it is important to have injuries treated. Neglected corneal injuries or infections may penetrate through the cornea into the eyeball and this can lead to loss of sight or necessitate surgical removal of the eyeball.

The majority of corneal injuries respond well to treatment, and after initial veterinary care, home treatment with dispensed eye ointments is all that is needed. If there is severe eye irritation, the dog may need to be kept in a darkened room for a few days.

CATARACT

The lens of the eye is a transparent capsule behind the pupil. Like the cornea, it has no blood supply and must remain clear or sight will be impaired. When the lens loses its transparency, the condition is called a cataract. There are many causes of cataracts, including congenital and inherited causes, trauma, radiation, eye injury, eye infections and secondary causes related to other diseases such as diabetes, and to old age (senile cataracts).

SYMPTOMS The pupil area will appear white if the whole lens is affected. If a dog is going blind from the development of cataracts, changes in behavior and bumping into objects in unfamiliar surroundings will occur.

DIAGNOSIS Diagnosis of a cataract is made by a veterinary physical examination of the eye.

TREATMENT There is no known medical treatment for a cataract. Many dogs get along very well with cataracts and retain a good deal of peripheral vision, but if the dog is going blind, surgical removal of the lens is the only treatment to restore the dog's vision.

A thorough physical and a detailed eye examination are essential prior to deciding on cataract surgery; there is no use proceeding if the retina has already been destroyed by some other disease process, and the dog is blind. The age and physical condition of the dog must also be taken into account. The surgery should be performed by a veterinary ophthalmologist if possible. Following removal of the lens, dogs can see quite adequately, as all they lose is the ability to focus and this ability is not well developed in the dog in any case. Therefore, unlike humans, dogs do not need to be fitted with glasses following lens removal!

The postsurgical period is critical following any eye surgery in dogs, as the surgeon's fine work can be quickly ruined if the dog scratches or rubs the eye. The eye is usually bandaged for protection and a special restraint collar may be required in dogs that tend to be self-mutilating. Most dogs will be kept in the veterinary hospital for a week or two following cataract surgery for these reasons, since it is very difficult for the owner to keep a close watch on the dog at all times.

PROGNOSIS Most dog owners are extremely pleased with the results of cataract surgery on their dog. Only a small percentage of cases turn out unsuccessfully for one reason or another. Even when the surgery proves unsuccessful, most dog owners feel they have done their duty, since their dogs were already blind and therefore not disadvantaged further by trying surgery.

Occasionally a dog that has been blind due to cataracts will get a return of vision if the lens breaks up and light can again enter the eye. This is called second sight.

Old-Age Eye Changes

As dogs age, the pupil will develop a blue gray appearance called nuclear sclerosis. In this condition the lens fibers increase in density and lose water, so that some of the light reaching the pupil is reflected back, giving the appearance of a cataract. However, when the eye is examined with an ophthalmoscope, nuclear sclerosis can be readily distinguished from a cataract. The dog retains good vision despite the appearance of the pupil. True senile cataracts do occur in old dogs, but in these cases, there is loss of vision.

GLAUCOMA

Glaucoma is an eye disease caused by an increase in pressure within the eye, arising from a restriction of the flow of fluid out of the eye or the production of too much fluid. The increased pressure inside the eye damages the optic nerve and other structures within the eye.

SYMPTOMS The external signs of glaucoma in the dog are a red, enlarged eye, pain, a cloudy cornea, dilation of the pupil with no response to light, and loss of vision. As glaucoma can lead to irreversible blindness in a few days, immediate treatment should be sought if any of these signs are seen in a dog.

DIAGNOSIS Diagnosis is made by symptoms and a veterinary eye examination. Further diagnostic signs will be evident to the veterinarian following tonometer pressure measurements and other specialized eye examinations.

TREATMENT Early treatment is essential to prevent blindness. Medical treatment is possible in most cases, but the drugs must be given daily by mouth, as well as medication applied to the eye itself. The drugs lower the pressure within the eye and prevent blindness, but they must be continued indefinitely. Follow-up medical check-ups by the veterinarian are essential, as changes in dosages or drugs will be needed to ensure that pain is controlled, the pressure is reduced, and the sight is maintained.

Three types of drugs are used to treat glaucoma: drugs that decrease the aqueous humor production; those that increase the outflow of aqueous humor; and those that decrease the intraocular volume.

Surgical treatment to reduce the pressure is used in selected cases where the dog owner cannot medicate the dog daily or the pressure cannot be reduced by medical treatment. If glaucoma cannot be controlled with treatment, the eye may have to be removed surgically.

RETINAL DISEASES

The retina is the light-receiving inner coat at the back of the eye. There are a number of retinal diseases and disorders that affect dogs, but these are not discussed in detail here because few respond to treatment and most lead to blindness. However, dogs manage very well if blind, provided they are allowed to live routine lives in familiar surroundings. Because of their highly developed senses of smell and hearing, they compensate for the blindness much better than their owners could.

The most common causes of retinal diseases in dogs are: congenital defects; injury to the eyes; eye infections and inflammations; blood vessel disorders of the eyes; detachment of the retina; tumors; vitamin deficiencies; and progressive retinal atrophy, which is an hereditary degeneration of the retina.

Many of the retinal diseases that occur in dogs are hereditary, so affected dogs should not be bred and should preferably be castrated or spayed.

6

The Ears

Ear disease in dogs is second only to skin disease in the number of cases seen yearly by veterinarians. A knowledge of the structure of a dog's ear is helpful in understanding why dogs have so many ear problems. The ear is made up of three parts: the external ear, composed of the earlobe, or earflap, and external ear canal; the middle ear, which includes an eardrum, an air cavity, and an auditory canal that connects with the nose and throat; and the inner ear, which houses the organs of hearing and equilibrium.

By far the greatest number of ear diseases and problems in dogs involve the external ear. Such conditions will often extend into the middle and inner ears if left untreated.

EXTERNAL EAR DISEASE (OTITIS EXTERNA)

Inflammation of the ear is called otitis. Technically, otitis externa is an inflammation of the external ear, but the term is more commonly used to refer specifically to inflammation of the external ear canal. The external ear canal in dogs is long and narrow, and in breeds with heavy hanging earflaps, these two anatomical arrangements prevent good air circulation, which leads to a moist ear that is more susceptible to inflam-

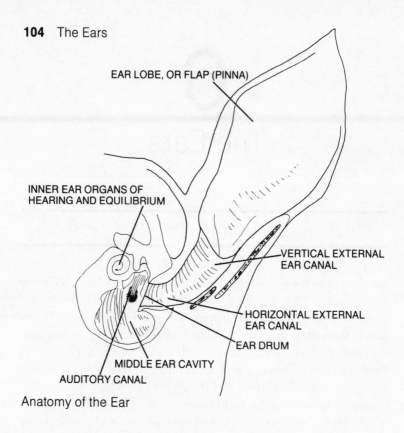

EAR LOBE, OR FLAP (PINNA)

INNER EAR ORGANS OF
HEARING AND EQUILIBRIUM

VERTICAL EXTERNAL
EAR CANAL

HORIZONTAL EXTERNAL
EAR CANAL

EAR DRUM

MIDDLE EAR CAVITY
AUDITORY CANAL

Anatomy of the Ear

mation and infection. Excessive hair in the ear canal in some
breeds also results in moist ears.

Otitis externa has numerous causes, including anything
that results in irritation to the external ear canal, such as
allergies; excessive earwax; excessive moisture in the ear;
bacterial infections (most commonly staphylococcal or streptococcal organisms); fungal infections, such as yeasts and
ringworm; parasitic mites or ticks; injuries; foreign bodies,
such as grass awns; tumors; poor ear drainage; infections
spreading from other areas of the body via the bloodstream;
hormone imbalances; vitamin deficiencies; and some skin diseases.

SYMPTOMS The inside of a dog's ear is normally light pink

in color and appears dry; when ear infections are present the lining of the ear appears wet, swollen, red, and sometimes ulcerated. Crusts and brownish or pus-like discharges may be seen, and the odor is frequently offensive. If the condition has been present for some time, the lining of the ear will be thickened and tough, and no discharge may be present. As any ear disease in dogs is painful and irritating, pawing at the ear, shaking the head, and scratching the ear are the most obvious diagnostic signs to both the owner and the veterinarian.

Otitis externa is frequently caused by ear mites and in these instances a black dry coating can be seen in the ear canal.

DIAGNOSIS   Otitis externa in dogs is diagnosed by the history, the clinical signs, a veterinary physical examination of the ear, and tests on the discharges or debris present in the ear canal. If some of this material is removed, ear mites, if present, can be observed with a magnifying glass as white moving specks among the black debris. They are even more visible under a microscope. Ticks also invade dogs' ears, but these are readily visible to the naked eye.

If parasites are not causing the dog's ear problem, the veterinarian will need to examine the ear canal with an otoscope (an instrument for inspecting the ear) and depending on the dog's temperament, this may require the use of a tranquilizer or even full anesthesia. A sample of the discharges will be examined under a microscope, which will reveal the cause of the ear problem in most instances. If the cause is a bacterial or fungal infection, a culture of the organism will need to be grown, and then sensitivity testing will be done to determine which drugs will be effective in treatment. Occasionally, a biopsy or surgical exploration will be needed to make a diagnosis. In long-standing or neglected cases it may not be possible to determine the cause, but in most acute ear problems a diagnosis can be made.

TREATMENT   Because veterinary practitioners see so many cases of otitis externa in dogs, they often treat them initially without conducting all these tests in order to save their clients added expenses. This is called diagnostic treatment, but if it is not successful, then diagnostic tests will be essential.

Treatment of otitis involves cleaning out the ear canal, preferably by the veterinarian with the dog sedated. Foreign bodies can then be readily seen and removed if they are the cause of the ear problem. Ointments containing antibiotics, cortisone, enzymes, insecticides, mineral oil, or wax-dissolving products are then used for follow-up treatment. Acute cases may require antibiotics by injection or by mouth. Tranquilizers, pain killers, and a restraint collar may be required in dogs that continue to mutilate their ears by scratching. If ear mites are the problem, other pets in the household will need to be checked and treated if infected, and a flea spray or powder will be recommended for the dog, other pets, and the pets' quarters.

PROGNOSIS The most common cause of failure in treatment of ear disease in dogs is inadequate home follow-up treatment; most often, the owner stops the ear or oral medication prematurely. This results in a relapse in many cases and can lead to a chronic condition. Failure also results if the medication is ineffective, so if there is no response to treatment in a few days, the dog owner should contact the veterinarian. Each time an infection recurs or is inadequately treated, the ear canal thickens and becomes narrower, and successful treatment by medication is more difficult. Surgical treatment involving partial or complete removal of the ear canal will then be the only approach available to cure the problem.

MIDDLE EAR DISEASE (OTITIS MEDIA)

Otitis media, an inflammation of the middle ear, is not encountered as frequently as otitis externa in dogs. In most cases, it is due to an extension of an external ear infection to the middle ear. Other infections can spread to the middle ear, particularly those of the nose and throat. Less common causes are perforation of the eardrum by a foreign body in the ear canal and tumors.

SYMPTOMS As most middle ear inflammations occur together with an external ear infection the signs are similar to those of otitis externa. However, middle ear infections are quite painful, so affected dogs are reluctant to move their heads. As a result there is less head shaking and scratching than in otitis externa alone. The head is often tilted down to the side of the affected ear and the earflap is also held down in dogs with erect ears. Depression, fever, and obvious pain on touching or moving the head are other accompanying signs of otitis media.

If not treated, otitis media can lead to serious complications, such as inner ear infections, osteomyelitis (bone infection) of the skull, meningitis, and brain abscess.

DIAGNOSIS The diagnosis is made from the history, symptoms, and a veterinary physical examination. An ear examination, usually under anesthesia, and x-rays are used to confirm the diagnosis. The further diagnostic approaches used in otitis externa are also applied in otitis media.

TREATMENT Treatment is the same as for otitis externa, but is more extensive and prolonged. Antibiotics will be required for up to four weeks, and pain-relieving drugs may also be needed for extended periods. If there is no response to treatment, then a myringotomy (a surgical incision of the eardrum) will be necessary to flush out the middle ear and allow the infection to drain.

PROGNOSIS Most cases respond well to treatment. The eardrum, whether perforated by a foreign body, as a result of infection, or surgically, heals in most cases. However, the dog's hearing does not appear to be affected even if the eardrum does not reform.

INNER EAR DISEASE (OTITIS INTERNA)

Otitis interna, inflammation of the inner ear, is a serious medical problem. Fortunately, it is rare in dogs. When it does occur, it is most commonly caused by an extension of an external and middle ear infection. Sometimes it occurs alone and in these instances the cause is usually from head trauma or a tumor. Long-term or excessive use of some antibiotics can sometimes lead to inner ear disease and hearing loss.

SYMPTOMS   The inner ear contains the organs of hearing and equilibrium, and symptoms are related to disease of these organs. Disturbed equilibrium is shown by abnormal posture and movement, including staggering, falling, and rolling movements, tilting of the head to the affected side, and circling to the affected side. A characteristic rapid movement of the eyeball, called nystagmus, is seen in most cases of otitis interna. Vomiting is another sign seen in severe cases. Behavior changes in the dog can indicate gradual or sudden deafness.

Inner ear infections may extend into the brain, causing meningitis and brain abscess, which can be fatal.

DIAGNOSIS   Diagnosis of otitis interna is made by the clinical signs and a veterinary physical examination. X-rays may be necessary to confirm the diagnosis. Many brain diseases and disorders have similar signs, so a diagnosis of otitis interna can be difficult to make unless the condition is accompanied by signs of xternal and middle ear disease. Tests for deafness will also be helpful diagnostically.

TREATMENT   If treated early, most cases respond to antibiotics and rest. Surgery can be done on the inner ear if other treatments fail, but it does not always have a successful outcome.

PROGNOSIS   Some dogs, despite a good response to treatment, will be left with permanent damage, such as a head tilt or deafness. Others will fail to respond and the outcome will be fatal.

EAR MITES

Ear mites are a common cause of otitis externa in dogs. The microscopic, eight-legged mites called *Otodectes cynotis* spend their entire lives on the dog, mainly in the ears, and live only a few days if separated from their host. They are transmitted from dog to dog, or cat, by direct contact. Ear mites, unlike sarcoptic mites, do not burrow into the skin, but live on the surface, where they puncture the skin of the ear canal and feed by sucking up lymph. This damages the lining of the ear canal, causes crusts to form, and eventually leads to bacterial infection of the ear canal. The entire life cycle of the mite—eggs, larvae, nymphs, adults—takes three to four weeks.

Complications of untreated ear mite infestations are the spread of the otitis to the middle or inner ears, and ear hematomas from scratching the earlobes.

Ear Mite (Enlarged)

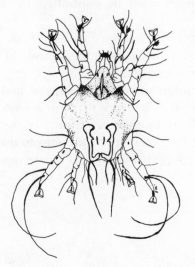

SYMPTOMS   Ear mites cause intense itching, and as a result of this irritation, the dog scratches the ears and shakes its head. The hair behind the ear or on the earflap may be scratched away, and the intense scratching can also lead to hematomas (bleeding beneath the skin) of the earflap. A dark brown-to-black debris inside the dog's ear is usually seen if ear mites are present.

DIAGNOSIS   The diagnosis of ear mites is made by the history, symptoms, and a veterinary physical examination of the ear. The mites can be seen in some of the discharge from the ear; they appear as moving white specks among the blackish debris. They are readily visible under the microscope.

TREATMENT   Treatment is the same as that for otitis externa and involves cleaning out the ear canal and the use of a miticide (insecticide to kill mites) in the ear. The miticide must be used for three to four weeks, twice a week. It kills the adult mites quickly, but those that are in the development stages are not as readily destroyed; treatment for one month is required to allow all the eggs to develop to adults and then be destroyed. If the ear is infected, antibiotic ointments may also be required. Corticosteroids are used if the intense irritation and scratching cannot be controlled by other treatments.

A flea spray or powder is necessary to kill any mites that escape from the ears. Other pets in the household should be checked and treated if infected.

PROGNOSIS   Ear mites are readily destroyed, and if the secondary ear infection is not severe or there are no complications, such as middle or internal ear infections, the prognosis is good—providing the dog owner continues to use the miticide for a long enough period to prevent recurrence of the ear mites.

EAR CLEANING AND HAIR REMOVAL

Dogs seldom need to have their ears cleaned because the natural wax secreted in the ears maintains healthy ear tissues. Excessive cleaning removes this wax, which can lead to tissue damage and even ear infections. However, if the ears are dirty or an infection is being treated, then cleaning can be helpful.

To clean a dog's ear, wrap a clean cloth around the index finger, dip it in water or mineral oil, and then insert the finger into the ear canal. Gently wipe the surfaces of the ear lining. A cotton-tipped swab dipped in mineral oil can be used to reach into the crevices.

The ear canal in the dog drops straight down and then takes a sharp turn inward toward the head, ending at the eardrum. As long as the swab is directed straight down, the dog

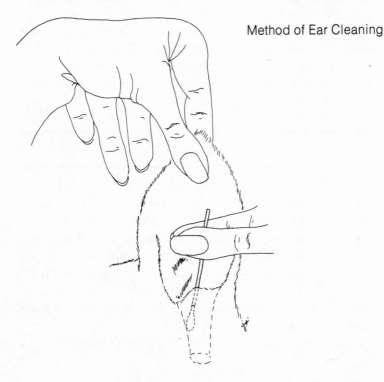

Method of Ear Cleaning

owner shouldn't damage the eardrum. In dogs with drooping ears, hold the earflap straight up while cleaning the canal, as this helps to straighten out the canal. Do not go too deeply into the ear because this may push the dirt further into the canal. Also, clean the inside of the earflaps as they may be the source of the dirt.

Poodles and terrier-type dogs often have excessive hair growing in the ear canal, which prevents good air circulation and makes them prone to ear problems. Many dog owners, groomers, and breeders pluck this hair out, but if not done properly it can lead to tissue damage and even more ear problems. Grasp the hair with the fingers or a tweezers and pull out with a sharp movement. Most dogs tolerate this well if it is done quickly and routinely. Do not irritate the ears or pull on hair that does not come out readily. Veterinarians prefer to clip the hair out as this causes less irritation, but it is difficult to do unless the dog is sedated.

When bathing a dog it is advisable to put cotton in its ears, because moisture in the ears sets up a condition that can eventually lead to infection. Another good preventive measure is to put cotton in a dog's ears when taking it through countryside that has vegetation or ticks that might get into the ears.

EAR SURGERY

In chronic cases of otitis externa or media, surgical reconstruction of the ear is recommended to expose the ear canal, thereby keeping the ear dry and aiding drainage—both of which promote healing. There are two types of surgery performed for this purpose. Lateral ear resection involves the removal of the outer wall of the ear canal and is by far the most common. Ablation of the ear canal involves complete removal of the ear canal and is used in very severe cases or if a tumor is present in the ear canal.

The response to either surgery is usually excellent, although it does take some time for full recovery because the ear tissues do not heal rapidly. The otitis will still need continuing treatment until the infection is fully cleared up.

EAR HEMATOMA

If there is bleeding under the skin of the earlobe or pinna, it is referred to as an ear hematoma. The most common causes are accidents or self-inflicted damage from the dog scratching the earlobe or violently shaking the head. Floppy-eared dogs are more often affected.

SYMPTOMS   A hematoma of the earlobe appears as a soft, fluctuating swelling from the localized accumulation of blood under the skin, and is readily visible.

TREATMENT   Many ear hematomas respond well to draining off the blood with a syringe and the application of a special ear support. However, some hematomas tend to reform, and in these cases a surgical procedure that involves incising the hematoma, draining the blood, and inserting special sutures may be needed. Postoperative care may require sedation and an Elizabethan collar restraint, to prevent the dog from reinjuring the ear. Hematomas can heal without any treatment, but usually this results in scarring and disfigurement of the ear lobe.

DEAFNESS

Deafness is not a common problem in dogs, nor is it easy to diagnose, as dogs tend to compensate well with their other senses. Temporary deafness may be caused by an infection, but hearing usually returns when the infection clears up. Senility, however, may be accompanied by permanent deafness. Deafness in dogs may be acquired or congenital (present from birth). Common causes of acquired deafness are ear infections, causing blockage of the ear canals; loud noises; trauma or infection of the inner ear; tumors of the inner ear or brain; certain diseases, such as canine distemper; long-term or excessive use of certain drugs, such as streptomycin, neomycin, and salicylates; and old age.

Congenital deafness is due to developmental defects of the hearing organs or nerves. Deafness due to an hereditary defect is more prevalent in white-haired dogs.

A punctured eardrum does not cause deafness, and in most instances, a perforated eardrum heals.

SYMPTOMS If a dog is going deaf, the owner will usually notice changes in behavior, including confusion, a failure to respond to verbal commands, and a lack of movement of the ear lobes. If a dog is born deaf, it is more difficult to see obvious signs of deafness because the dog learns to compensate so well with its other senses. A lack of response to a loud noise that awakens and disturbs a dog with normal hearing is the clearest sign of deafness.

DIAGNOSIS Diagnosis of deafness is made by the history, symptoms, and a veterinary physical examination. Testing the reaction of the dog to noise stimuli, an examination of the ears, x-rays, and a neurological examination may all be required to diagnose deafness in a dog. In acquired deafness, the cause can usually be determined, but in congenital deafness all structures and functions may appear normal—except that the dog cannot hear.

TREATMENT In acquired deafness, removal of the cause will often reverse the deafness, particularly if the deafness is due to blockage of the external or middle ears from otitis. Congenital deafness can seldom be reversed, and such dogs should not be bred because the deafness may be an inherited defect.

EAR CROPPING

Ear cropping involves the surgical removal of a portion of each earlobe in order to make the ears stand erect. It is done purely for cosmetic reasons to conform with the standards set for these breeds. The surgery is done at a critical age in the dog's development and can leave psychological scars. The postsurgical period is, at least, uncomfortable for the puppy, if not painful; it also involves taping and splinting the ears. If the ears do not stand correctly, the tapes and splints are often required for weeks.

The breeds that have their ears cropped are Doberman pinschers, Great Danes, boxers, schnauzers, Boston terriers, Manchester terriers, Bouvier des Flandres, and Brussels griffons. Cropping is usually done between seven and ten weeks of age, except in Boston terriers, which are cropped between four and six months of age.

Although a formal survey has not been conducted among veterinarians concerning ear cropping and their attitude to it, the decision appears to be split as to the value of such surgeries. Many veterinarians who do not approve of these procedures still perform them because they can do the job with professional skill.

In the past, ear cropping was done to prevent hunting dogs from having their ears torn by thorny bushes. Today, however, pet dogs are seldom exposed to such hazards, and ear cropping is done for purely aesthetic reasons.

Ear cropping has been illegal in England since 1895—a humane and civilized law. It is to be hoped that dog owners, dog breeders, and veterinarians in the United States will eventually unite to change the standards for the affected breeds so that this unnecessary surgery can be eliminated.

7

The Teeth

Many dog owners do not realize that dogs need dental care. In fact, however, dogs suffer from all the same dental problems that people do, including: plaque and tartar build-up, dental caries (cavities), tooth root abscesses, gingivitis (inflammation of the gums), periodontitis (inflammation of the structures around the tooth), retained deciduous teeth, malocclusions (bad bite), and tumors of the teeth and gums. Routine care of the teeth in dogs, both by the owner daily and the veterinarian once a year, can prevent most of these dental problems, save the dog from pain and unnecessary tooth loss, and save the owner the expense of special dental treatments.

DENTAL ANATOMY OF THE DOG

Number of Teeth

Dogs have twenty-eight deciduous (temporary or primary) teeth and forty-two permanent teeth, versus twenty and thirty-two respectively for humans. Dogs are born with no teeth, and the deciduous teeth start to appear at two to three weeks of age and begin to be replaced by the permanent teeth at fourteen to sixteen weeks of age. All the permanent teeth have appeared by eight months of age.

Adult dogs have the following teeth:

Teeth	Upper Jaw	Lower Jaw
Incisors	6	6
Canines	2	2
Premolars	8	8
Molars	4	6
TOTAL:	20	22

Dog owners often ask veterinarians to tell them how old a dog is by looking at its teeth. An estimate can be made of the age of a dog by the amount of wear and the condition of the teeth, but this is by no means accurate after the dog is eight months old.

Anatomy of the Tooth

The tooth is made up of the crown, which is the visible portion that ends at the gumline, and the root(s), which are below the gumline and embedded in the bones of the jaws. The tooth itself has three layers. The outer layer of the crown is covered with enamel, which is the hardest substance in the body. In the root area the enamel is replaced by cementum. The middle layer of the crown and the root is made up of dentin, which is harder than bone, but not as hard as enamel.

Section of a Tooth

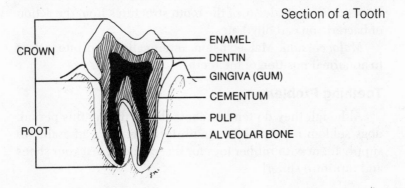

CROWN

ROOT

— ENAMEL
— DENTIN
— GINGIVA (GUM)
— CEMENTUM
— PULP
— ALVEOLAR BONE

The inner core, or center, of the tooth in the crown and root areas contains pulp, consisting of nerve, blood, and other structural tissues.

Dental Terms

The following medical words are used frequently when discussing dental problems:

Periodontal. Literally translated, periodontal means "around the tooth" and refers to the structures which suspend the tooth in the jaw. These structures include the gingiva, which is the gum; a ligament which extends between the cementum of the root and the bone of the root socket; and the alveolar bone, which is the cavity or socket in the jawbone in which the roots of the teeth are attached.

Gingiva. Gingiva is a technical word for the gums.

Dental plaque. Dental plaque is a white filmy substance which deposits mainly at the gum margins of the teeth. It is made up of food debris, epithelial cells (gum cells), saliva components, and bacteria (most commonly streptococcal organisms).

Tartar, or dental calculus. When dental plaque becomes mineralized with calcium salts it forms hard yellow-to-brownish or black deposits on the teeth. These are referred to as calculus or tartar.

Dental caries. Dental caries are commonly called cavities. (Caries means decay.) Dental caries is a disease of the teeth in which there is decay of the tooth structures from the action of bacteria on carbohydrates.

Malocclusion. Malocclusion, often called bad bite, refers to abnormal position of the teeth.

Teething Problems

Although they do tend to chew things during this period, dogs seldom have problems with teething. It is advisable to supply them with rubber toys for this purpose, lest your shoes and furniture suffer!

Occasionally a deciduous tooth is retained or not shed, and this can prevent the permanent tooth from coming up. If a tooth is retained past eight months of age, it should be removed, providing that a check has revealed that a permanent tooth replacement is present.

The presence of supernumerary (extra) teeth is not an uncommon occurrence in dogs. However, these extra teeth should be removed, since they often lead to crowding of the other teeth, malocclusion (or bad bite), and periodontitis (inflammation of tissues).

Discolored teeth or teeth that are pitted can result from severe diseases, nutritional deficiencies, or parasites affecting the puppy during the first two months of life, when the teeth are developing. Certain drugs administered during this period can also cause these teeth defects. By and large, discolored or pitted teeth do not present a medical problem.

MALOCCLUSION (TEETH POSITION ABNORMALITIES)

Any condition in which the teeth are not normally positioned is called a malocclusion. Abnormalities of bite are relatively common in dogs. Undershot jaw (lower jaw protrudes beyond the upper jaw) is seen and is normal in breeds such as pugs and bulldogs. Overshot jaw (upper jaw protrudes beyond the lower jaw) also occurs and is familiarly known as buck teeth. Unless the malocclusion is causing a problem it is not necessary to interfere surgically.

TARTAR (DENTAL CALCULUS)

Tartar, also known as dental calculus, is made up of calcium salts, food debris, bacteria, and other organic matter. It is yellow-to-brownish, or black in color and develops from soft dental plaque that becomes mineralized with calcium salts and hardens into tartar. It collects primarily on the cheek side of the upper premolars and molars. Dental tartar is seen mostly in dogs over six years of age, or in younger dogs that eat only soft foods.

SYMPTOMS The tartar deposits can be readily seen on examining the dog's teeth. Tartar is usually accompanied by gingivitis (inflammation of the gums) and periodontitis (inflammation of the tissues around the tooth). Without treatment, the teeth will loosen and fall out.

TREATMENT If the calculus is not too severe and if the dog is cooperative, your veterinarian may be able to remove the tartar build-up without sedation, or with the use of a tranquilizer. In order to do a professional job, however, it is necessary to anesthetize the dog. The tartar can then be removed, the teeth can be scaled and cleaned, and the gums treated where necessary (*see* Periodontitis, later in this chapter).

PREVENTION There are a number of methods of preventing tartar accumulation on dogs' teeth. Feeding dry dog food or hard dog biscuits helps reduce the build-up of tartar. Allowing dogs to chew on large, hard bones is also effective, but is not without some hazard because dogs will invariably chip off and swallow bone fragments that can cause constipation or a life-threatening bowel blockage or rupture. Hard rubber toys are less effective in preventing tartar accumulation, but are safer—provided they are large enough so that they cannot be swallowed by the dog accidentally. Another useful product to help keep a dog's teeth clean is the rawhide bone or toy. These products, available from pet stores and many supermarkets, will keep a dog happily occupied for hours and also distract it from chewing your furniture and personal belongings.

Wiping the dog's teeth daily with a saline (salt) solution (½ teaspoon salt to 1 cup of warm water) is an effective way to prevent tartar accumulation. The really conscientious dog owner will brush the dog's teeth daily with special toothbrushes and toothpastes now available from veterinarians. Baking soda is a good dentifrice to use on dogs' teeth as dogs do not object too much to the taste, and it will not harm them if they swallow it. Many dog owners think brushing their dogs' teeth is going a bit too far, but those who make this kind of effort save themselves the expense and inconvenience of having to take their dog to the veterinarian for frequent teeth scaling and cleaning. Such dogs also do not have to suffer the pain and discomfort that accompanies tartar build-up. Additionally, gum infections and loss of teeth, which can eventually occur if tartar is neglected, can be avoided. Water flushing is also an effective method of keeping a dog's teeth clean and can be done with an electric Water Pik, a syringe, a hose, or even a water pistol.

A once-a-year cleaning by your veterinarian is recommended, starting at eighteen months of age.

DENTAL CARIES (TOOTH CAVITIES)

Dental caries, or tooth cavities, are not as rare in dogs as many dog owners or even veterinarians suggest. In a recent study, it was found that 10% of dogs aged three to seven years had one or more cavities. The incidence in dogs is not as high as that in people, probably because dogs do not normally consume a lot of sugars. In dogs, the cavities tend to appear at or below the gum and tooth margin; in people, most cavities appear on the crown of the teeth. Because of the gum-margin position of cavities in dogs, the decay is much faster, and harder to detect.

Dental cavities are formed by the action of the bacteria on food debris, both of which are present in dental plaque. Streptococcal bacteria and other organisms act on food carbohydrates to form lactic acid, and this acid decalcifies or breaks down the enamel or cementum layer of the tooth. This results in a soft, chalky white spot on the tooth, which later becomes stained and dark colored. Eventually the decay invades the dentin layer of the tooth and enters the pulp cavity.

SYMPTOMS   Very often there are no signs of dental caries in dogs, and the cavities are difficult to observe because of their location at or below the gumline. If the cavities are advanced or the tooth becomes abscessed, signs of mouth pain, reluctance to chew, increased salivation, and pawing at the mouth will be evident.

DIAGNOSIS   The diagnosis of tooth cavities in dogs is made by a veterinary physical examination of the mouth using a dental probe and can be confirmed by x-rays if necessary. The dog may have to be sedated or anesthetized for a complete mouth examination, but in most instances, tartar accumulation and periodontitis will also be evident and will need treatment. In this event, examination for cavities will be done during treatment.

TREATMENT   There are three approaches to tooth cavities in dogs, and the choice will depend on the severity of the decay, the tooth involved, and on how much the dog owner wishes to spend on trying to save the tooth.

Extraction. If the decay is advanced, the veterinarian will usually recommend extraction of the tooth.

Filling the cavity. If the decay is not too far advanced, the decay can be removed and a restorative material such as an amalgam or resin can be inserted in the cavity. Many veterinarians do not do this dental work themselves and may refer the dog owner to another practitioner who does such work as a special interest, or they may call in a dentist as a consultant.

Endodontic or root canal treatment. Endodontic means within the tooth, and endodontics is dentistry which deals with the diagnosis and treatment of pulp tissue problems. If a tooth cavity has spread to the pulp, then a root canal will be required. This involves removal of the pulp, cleaning out the pulp chamber or canal, inserting a filling material into the canal, and then sealing the area with amalgam or resin. Root canal work is now being done on occasion in dogs, but it is expensive and usually requires a dentist as a consultant, so dog owners seldom request this specialized dentistry. Root canal treatment is used quite often in dogs if they break off one of their canine teeth, since part of the tooth can then be saved, and the trauma and pain of extraction can be avoided. In some cases a cap has been made to replace the missing portion of the tooth.

PERIODONTITIS (PERIODONTAL DISEASE)

Periodontitis, also called pyorrhea, is an inflammation of the structures around the tooth. These structures include the gums, the periodontal ligament between the tooth root and the bone of the socket, the cementum, which is the outer layer of the root, and the alveolar bone, which is the tooth socket bone around the root of the tooth. Inflammation of the gums is called gingivitis.

Periodontal disease develops over a number of years, with the build-up of dental plaque (a white filmy substance that accumulates at the gum and teeth margins and is made up of food debris, epithelial cells, saliva components, and bacteria). The bacteria gain access to the gums at the teeth margins, which causes inflammation of the gums. This inflammation then spreads to the tissues around each tooth root or socket; this condition is referred to as periodontitis. The condition, if not treated, progresses to loss of bone around the teeth sockets and loosening of the teeth. The gums then recede and the teeth eventually fall out. The complete process is called periodontal disease. Further complicating this disease is the formation of tartar, or dental calculus, from the dental plaque as it becomes mineralized with calcium salts. The tartar forms on the sides of the teeth and to a degree even below the gumline, so it also contributes to the inflammation and irritation of the gums.

Periodontitis is present in about 85% of dogs over six years of age in the United States. A soft diet is a contributing factor, but without dental care, all dogs will be affected as they get older.

Complications that can arise from periodontitis are a tooth abscess, a bone infection of the jaw, and if the bacteria enter the bloodstream, a septicemia (blood poisoning), or even heart disease.

Other causes of periodontitis are injury or trauma to the mouth; malocclusion; foreign bodies in the mouth, such as foxtails and porcupine quills; vitamin deficiencies, especially of the B vitamins; low calcium levels in the blood; heavy metal (such as lead) poisonings; diabetes mellitus; generalized body infections; chronic kidney or other debilitating diseases; and leukemias.

SYMPTOMS Periodontitis is a slowly developing disease in most dogs, so the signs will vary depending on its severity and extent. The early signs are plaque deposits and red and swollen gums which may bleed readily. Later signs include tartar deposits, a foul odor to the breath, loosening of the teeth, and even loss of some teeth. If the gums are infected, pus may be seen at the gum and teeth margins.

In advanced periodontal disease, particularly if complicated by an abscess or dental caries, the dog will be reluctant to chew and will exhibit pain if the mouth is touched. In some advanced cases the dog may refuse to eat at all, and depression and fever may also be evident.

DIAGNOSIS The diagnosis is made by the symptoms and a veterinary physical examination. X-rays and a dental probe examination of the mouth under anesthesia may be required to determine the extent and severity of the disease.

TREATMENT In most cases, periodontitis will clear up once the condition causing it has been treated. Removal of the dental plaque and tartar by scaling, cleaning, and polishing the teeth is all that is needed in most instances. Scaling can be done with mechanical ultrasonic or air turbine scaler equipment, or manually using special instruments designed for this purpose. In order for your veterinarian to do a thorough job, the dog will need to be sedated and given local anesthetics, or fully anesthetized if extensive treatment is required. If there is severe gum disease, the infected gum tissue will need to be surgically excised. Loose teeth will be extracted, and decayed teeth will be extracted, filled, or given root canal repair.

Antibiotics and vitamins, particularly the B-complex vitamins, may be required for follow-up treatment. Application of a saline solution or antiseptic to the gums for a few weeks may also be recommended; a saline solution of ½ teaspoon salt to 1 cup of warm water is used. If extensive mouth work was done, pain killers and a soft diet for a few days may be required.

Periodontal disease can be chronic in dogs with kidney failure and other incurable diseases. In these cases improvement can be affected with proper care, but the condition cannot be cured.

PREVENTION Periodontal disease can be prevented or kept to a minimum by the following measures (*see also* Tartar Prevention, above):

1. Cleaning the dog's teeth at least twice a week.
2. Feeding the dog a firm, fibrous diet, such as dry dog food and dog biscuits. Avoid a soft diet.
3. Having the dog's teeth routinely checked by your veterinarian, at least once a year. Have them scaled, cleaned, and polished, if recommended.

TOOTH ROOT ABSCESS

An abscess is a localized collection of pus in a cavity. When bacteria invade the pulp tissue and surrounding root tissues of a tooth, a tooth root abscess forms. The cause can be from the fracture of a tooth, extension of periodontal disease, dental caries, or an infection in another area of the body carried to the teeth by the bloodstream.

SYMPTOMS   A tooth root abscess causes pain, swelling of the face, excessive salivation, loss of appetite, depression, and fever. The abscess may drain into the mouth, or sometimes to the outside of the face or chin. The upper canine teeth often drain through the nose to the mouth. The fourth upper premolar may drain into the maxillary sinus below the eye, and then drain through the skin of the cheek. The lower teeth may drain through the skin of the lower jaw.

DIAGNOSIS   Diagnosis is by the symptoms and a physical examination of the mouth; it is confirmed by x-rays.

TREATMENT   Treatment requires surgical extraction of the affected tooth and drainage of the abscess. Antibiotics will be given to clear up the infection.

8

The Cardiovascular System

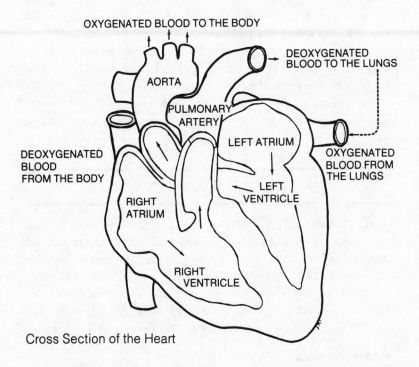

OXYGENATED BLOOD TO THE BODY

DEOXYGENATED
BLOOD TO THE LUNGS

AORTA

PULMONARY
ARTERY

LEFT ATRIUM

DEOXYGENATED
BLOOD
FROM THE BODY

OXYGENATED
BLOOD FROM
THE LUNGS

LEFT
VENTRICLE

RIGHT
ATRIUM

RIGHT
VENTRICLE

Cross Section of the Heart

HEART FUNCTION

The heart is a muscular pump with four chambers and sets of valves designed to circulate blood throughout the body tissues. The four sets of valves must open and shut in precise sequence to keep the blood pumping in one direction, carrying oxygen and nutrients to and wastes from the tissues.

The left side of the heart receives freshly oxygenated bright red blood from the lungs and pumps it out the aorta and throughout the arteries to the body tissues.

The blood returns to the right side of the heart from the body tissues via the veins; it is bluish in color because it has been depleted of oxygen. From the right side of the heart it is pumped to the lungs, where it exchanges carbon dioxide for oxygen. It is then returned to the left side of the heart to be pumped out to the body tissues.

The heartbeat is regulated by a special part of the heart called the pacemaker, which controls the heart rate and rhythm by emitting electrical impulses. The coronary arteries supply blood to the heart muscle; when one of these arteries blocks, a person is said to have had a coronary or a heart attack.

HEART DISEASE AND HEART FAILURE

There are many similarities between heart disease in dogs and humans. Although the human mortality rate from heart disease has been dropping in recent years, in dogs it is on the increase. In fact, 75% of dogs over nine years of age have some evidence of heart disease on postmortem examination. Despite these statistics, only about 25% of dogs with heart disease will actually show signs of heart failure in their lifetime.

Heart Disease

The most common causes of heart disease in dogs are:

Chronic valvular fibrosis. In this disease the valves of the heart become thickened and distorted, leaking when the heart contracts. This is the most frequent cause of heart failure in dogs.

Myocarditis and endocarditis. This is an inflammation of the heart muscle and lining of the heart, respectively. The usual cause is bacterial, viral, or fungal infection.

Heartworm disease. The heart is damaged by large worms, which lodge in the right side of the heart. Heartworm disease is transmitted by mosquitoes in infected areas.

Cardiac arrhythmias. These are changes in the normal rhythm of the heart and can lead to heart failure. Most heart disease will result in some type of arrhythmia, although not all arrhythmias indicate heart disease.

Cardiomyopathy. This is a condition in which the heart muscle is weakened, either by enlargement of the heart chambers or of the heart muscle itself.

Congenital problems. Congenital defects or malformations of the heart muscle, vessels, or valves.

Anemia.

High blood pressure.

Trauma.

Tumors.

Heart Failure

Whatever the cause of heart disease, heart failure is the final outcome when the disease becomes advanced. Heart failure is the inability of the heart to meet the oxygen demands of the body tissues, because a failing heart cannot pump the blood to all parts of the body adequately. To compensate for this failure, the heart muscle thickens and enlarges, and for a while the resultant increased cardiac output is adequate. The kidneys sense this heart failure and set up a protective mechanism by retaining salt and water which increases the circulating blood volume and thereby brings the cardiac output back to normal. Eventually, the failing heart can no longer handle this increased blood volume, and blood backs up. Fluid from the blood leaks into the body tissues and the lungs. This is edema, or swelling.

There are three types of heart failure:

1. *Right-sided.* If the right side of the heart fails, blood returning to the heart from throughout the body backs up, and fluid accumulation is most noticeable in the liver, abdomen, and limbs.

2. *Left-sided.* If the left side of the heart fails, blood returning from the lungs to the heart backs up, and fluid accumulates in the lungs.

3. *Right- and left-sided.* If both sides of the heart fail, the entire blood circulation system is affected.

SYMPTOMS   Although many dogs, particularly as they age, have heart disease, symptoms only become evident when the heart starts to fail. The signs depend on the severity of the disease and on which side of the heart is affected, and include some or all of the following:

- General weakness and fatigue, particularly noticeable after exercise. Some dogs may faint if forced to exercise.
- Shortness of breath and a cough, Most evident in left-sided heart failure, these are symptoms of an accumulation of fluid in the lungs.
- Swelling of the abdomen and limbs. Most evident in right-sided heart failure. This edema is due to an accumulation of fluid throughout the body. Pressure on the swollen feet will leave a deep indentation or depression that is slow to disappear; this condition is called pitting edema.
- A bluish appearance to the tongue and gums as a result of the poor blood circulation.
- A poor appetite and signs of digestive disturbances such as vomiting, diarrhea, or constipation. These may occur from inadequate blood circulation to the liver and digestive organs.
- Excessive drinking and urination.
- An increased heart rate and weak pulse.

DIAGNOSIS   A veterinarian can diagnose heart disease in a dog in most cases from the history, symptoms, and a physical examination. However, some or all of the following diagnostic procedures will be necessary to try to determine the cause and degree of heart failure. These procedures will assist the veterinarian in choosing the best method of treatment for a dog with heart failure.

Stethoscope examination. A stethoscope is an instrument used by all doctors to listen to the heart sounds and rhythms. Many dogs with heart disease have murmurs, which are abnormal sounds caused by turbulence of blood in a heart with leaky valves. Abnormal heart rate and abnormal breath sounds from fluid in the lungs will also be heard.

X-ray examination. X-rays will show changes in the size, shape, and position of the heart and evidence of fluid in the lungs.

Blood and urine tests. Blood tests are useful in determining many body functions and the presence of anemia. A specific blood test can be performed to diagnose heartworms in dogs. Urine tests are required to evaluate kidney function, which may be seriously impaired in heart failure.

Electrocardiogram (ECG). An electrocardiogram is a graphic recording or display of the electrical activity produced by the heart muscle and is a valuable diagnostic tool in heart disease. Nearly everyone has seen ECGs displayed on a screen in a TV medical program or in a hospital. More than 4,000 veterinary hospitals throughout the United States subscribe to a telephone ECG interpretation service that transmits the cardiogram by phone to a veterinary cardiologist for diagnosis, prognosis, and recommended treatments.

Cardiac catheterization. In this procedure, blood is withdrawn from the heart through a tube inserted into a front limb blood vessel. Analysis of the blood can be of diagnostic value in heart disease cases. This is not a routine procedure and is only done in selected cases of heart disease.

Angiocardiography. In this technique the course of dyes injected into the bloodstream can be traced through the heart and circulation by x-rays, and the results can be very informative on the function and structure of the heart. This procedure is not used routinely by veterinarians, as it is expensive to perform and can be hazardous.

Phonocardiography. This is a graphic recording of the sounds produced by the heart and can be useful in diagnosis.

Although some expense is involved in having these tests done on a dog with heart disease, it is money well spent because an accurate diagnosis is the key to effective treatment. Any treatment based on a misdiagnosis is worthless and expensive in the long run, and may even cost the dog its life in something as serious as heart disease.

TREATMENT   Treatment of heart failure in dogs is very similar to treatment of this condition in humans. In most cases it is not complicated and is very worthwhile. The objective of heart failure treatment is to balance the output of the heart and meet the tissues' oxygen needs, both of which are impaired in heart failure. Fortunately, there are many excellent drugs available today. The approaches to treatment are:

1. *Activity restriction.* Many dogs with heart failure will need to have their exercise restricted, and this can vary from minimal to severe restriction. Because dogs are not as cooperative as people, tranquilizers, sedatives, or enforced cage rest may be required.

2. *Low-sodium diets.* Salt restriction is essential in treating heart failure, because sodium chloride (salt) is retained by the body and this leads to edema (a build-up of water in the tissues). Specially formulated low-sodium diets, such as Prescription Diet h/d made by Hill's, are available from your veterinarian; however, dogs (like people) often find salt-free food unpalatable at first, so it may take some determination on the owner's part to make this essential changeover. A home-made diet can also be used (*see* Chapter 1, Nutrition; Types of Diets for Dogs: Heart Failure Diet). Water must never be restricted in dogs with heart failure, but softened water should be avoided, because it has a high salt content.

3. *Diuretics.* These are drugs used to stimulate kidney activity to remove retained water from the body via urination, which will be increased in amount and frequency.

4. *Digitalis.* This is a heart muscle stimulant; it improves cardiac output by increasing the force and decreasing the rate of contraction of the heart muscle.

5. *Other drugs.* There are many drugs available today for treating heart disease. Quinidine and propranolol are two used to smooth out or slow down irregular or fast heartbeats in dogs.

6. *Oxygen, bronchodilators, and cough suppressants.* Some or all of these may be needed in specific cases of heart failure to help the lungs function more efficiently.

7. *Heartworm disease medications.* Heartworm disease can be successfully treated by specific medications in most cases (*see* section later in this chapter). Preventive drugs to avoid reinfection are essential following treatment.

8. *Surgery.* Treatment of heart disease through surgery is not common in dogs, not because it cannot be done, but because of the expense. Some veterinary practitioners and all university small-animal veterinary departments perform surgeries in dogs for congenital defects of the heart, valve defects, heart injury from accidents, heartworm removal, insertion of electronic pacemakers, and even heart transplants.

Treatment of heart disease in dogs is not complicated or expensive after the initial diagnosis and treatment regimen have been established. Initial treatment may require the dog to be hospitalized to allow the veterinarian to monitor its response to treatment, and to determine the drugs needed for treatment and their most effective dosage level.

The prognosis in heart failure will depend on how early the dog is brought to the veterinarian for treatment and on the severity of the heart disease. The majority of dogs respond very well to treatment, and lead active, happy, and even long lives, quite often dying from old age or causes unrelated to heart failure. However, except in rare cases, heart failure is an incurable and progressive disease and will require treatment for the rest of the dog's life. Most dogs suffering from heart failure are older and have been with their owners a long time, and the emotional bonds between them are very strong. For these reasons the majority of such owners feel the treatment of heart failure is well worthwhile and are most grateful when they see their dog become happy and active again.

HIGH BLOOD PRESSURE (HYPERTENSION)

Dog owners often ask why veterinarians do not take a dog's blood pressure when they do a routine physical examination. Veterinarians would like to be able routinely to take blood pressure measurements in their canine patients, but unfortunately it is very difficult to get accurate blood pressure readings in dogs that have not been trained to accept the pressure cuff. There are several other methods of obtaining blood pressure readings in dogs, but most of them are only used during surgery, in cases of shock, and for certain types of heart disease.

Dogs do not suffer from high blood pressure (hypertension) to the same degree as people. In experimental studies in dogs, it has been found that dietary excesses, stress, and kidney disease can cause hypertension.

HEARTWORM DISEASE

Heartworm disease, also called Dirofilariasis, is caused by a worm scientifically named *Dirofilaria immitis*. These worms are found in the right side of the heart and in the large adjacent vessels. The female worm is 6 to 14 inches long and ⅛ inch wide—the male is smaller—and one dog may have as

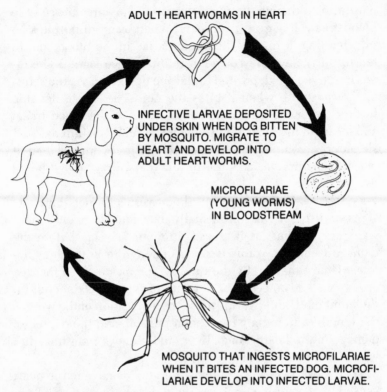

ADULT HEARTWORMS IN HEART

INFECTIVE LARVAE DEPOSITED
UNDER SKIN WHEN DOG BITTEN
BY MOSQUITO. MIGRATE TO
HEART AND DEVELOP INTO
ADULT HEARTWORMS.

MICROFILARIAE
(YOUNG WORMS)
IN BLOODSTREAM

MOSQUITO THAT INGESTS MICROFILARIAE
WHEN IT BITES AN INFECTED DOG. MICROFI-
LARIAE DEVELOP INTO INFECTED LARVAE.

Life Cycle of Heartworms

many as 300 worms. Heartworm disease is very serious and potentially fatal.

Heartworm disease in dogs occurs all over the world. In the United States, it was once limited to the South and Southeast regions, but has been spreading rapidly and is now found in most regions and in Canada, particularly where mosquitoes are prevalent. The disease is not spread directly from dog to dog, but requires an intermediate host, in this case a mosquito, for transmission.

Adult female worms produce millions of young immature worms called microfilariae, which live in the bloodstream. They cannot grow to maturity without first passing through a mosquito, although they can continue to circulate in the bloodstream for up to two years. When a mosquito bites an infected dog, it ingests the microfilariae in the blood, and in ten to thirty days they develop into infective larvae. The infective larvae are deposited under the dog's skin via the saliva of the mosquito when it bites the dog. The larvae develop further under the skin and eventually enter the bloodstream and locate in the heart. They become sexually mature in about six months, completing the life cycle of the worm. The adult worms can survive for three to ten years, the average being five years.

SYMPTOMS   Most dogs with heartworms do not show any signs of disease. Dogs are usually over four years old before signs are obvious, as it takes a number of years before the damage from the worms is severe enough to produce symptoms. Unfortunately, by the time symptoms are seen the disease is well advanced. The severity of symptoms depends on the number of adult worms present, the location of the worms, the length of time they have been present, and the degree of damage to the heart, lungs, liver, and kidneys from the adult worms and microfilariae.

The most obvious symptoms from the damage to the heart caused by the adult worms are a soft, dry chronic cough, shortness of breath, weakness, nervousness, loss of stamina, and listlessness. Advanced cases show more serious signs of heart failure.

The microfilariae primarily affect the small blood vessels (capillaries) of the lungs, liver, kidneys, and brain, and by their presence block the blood flow through these organs. The symptoms are related to disease in these organs and are manifested by coughing, jaundice, anemia, and general weakness.

DIAGNOSIS   In most cases, whether there are signs of disease or not, a diagnosis of heartworm disease can be made by a relatively simple blood test in which the microfilariae can be identified. If signs of heart failure are present, further diagnostic tests will be required to determine if the dog can tolerate treatment to destroy the heartworms, and also to determine if heart failure treatment will be required (*see* Diagnosis of Heart Disease, earlier in this chapter). Cases diagnosed early can usually be treated successfully, and the heart will not have been permanently damaged.

TREATMENT There is some risk in treating dogs with heartworms, but fatalities are rare. If the disease is very advanced it may be safer to just treat the heart failure and other symptoms, but this, of course, is a decision for the dog owner and veterinarian to make.

There is some controversy on the best method of treatment. The most accepted treatment is to give medication to kill the adult worms first and later treat to kill the microfilariae (young immature worms). The other treatment reverses this.

Adult worm treatment. Treatment to destroy the adult worms involves the injection of an arsenic drug into the bloodstream, usually four times over two days. Because arsenic is toxic not only to the heartworms but also to the dog, this treatment is performed while the dog is hospitalized. The adult worms die in a few days and start to decompose. This is a hazardous stage for the dog because the disintegrating worms are carried to the lungs and this can lead to respiratory problems. The worms are eventually reabsorbed, but dogs must be kept quiet and not allowed to exercise for one month following this treatment (when this process is occurring), and a cough may be noticeable for a few months. If a dog has a bad reaction in the weeks following the initial treatment and shows loss of appetite, shortness of breath, fever, and depression, the veterinarian will need to be notified, as supportive treatments may be necessary.

Microfilariae treatment. A number of drugs are available to kill the microfilariae. One of these drugs is used about six weeks after the treatment to kill the adult worms. The drug is given by mouth for one week, and the blood is then tested for the presence of microfilariae. If still positive, further seven-day treatments are repeated until the blood test is negative.

These drugs are also somewhat toxic, so if vomiting and weakness occur, it may be necessary to stop treatment and try again later.

Heart failure treatment. If signs of heart failure are present, treatment will be necessary (*see* Treatment of Heart Failure, earlier in this chapter).

Surgery. Heart surgery to remove the worms is another method of treatment, but it is usually reserved for special cases with advanced liver or kidney damage, or where the response to arsenic treatment was too severe. As these are the poor-risk patients, the survival rate is not good, but sometimes it is the only way to try to save the dog's life.

PROGNOSIS Most dogs respond very well to treatment, and those showing symptoms of disease prior to treatment have renewed vigor and vitality. However, despite these improvements, activity must be restricted for at least six weeks.

PREVENTION Dogs that have been treated for heartworms and dogs that test negative but live in heartworm disease areas must be given preventive treatment to avoid reinfection or infection. The drug used for prevention (diethylcarbamazine) destroys the infective larvae when they are deposited under the skin by an infected mosquito. The drug is available in pill, powder, or liquid form, and is given by mouth or added to the food. A special diet (Control Diet HRH made by Hill's) which contains the drug is now available. Preventive medication must be administered daily from just before the start of the mosquito season to two months after and all yearlong in the warmer, moist climates. The drug costs only a few cents a day and has the added advantage of also preventing and controlling roundworms and hookworms.

Caution: Twice-yearly blood tests are recommended to test for heartworms in dogs, because dogs must never be put on the preventive drug until the adult worms and microfilariae have been destroyed, or a severe and sometimes fatal reaction may occur.

Using screens and insecticides, and spraying mosquito

breeding grounds are helpful preventive measures, but 100% mosquito control is nearly impossible.

With regular blood testing of dogs, preventive treatment, and mosquito abatement, heartworm disease can be kept under control and may eventually be eliminated.

ANEMIA

Blood is a body tissue which circulates. It is made up of red blood cells, called erythrocytes; white blood cells, called leukocytes; plasma, which is the fluid portion of the blood; and other components, such as blood platelets, which are involved in blood clotting. The red blood cells are formed in the bone marrow and survive about three or four months. The hemoglobin in the red blood cells has the ability to pick up oxygen in the lungs and release it to the body tissues, where it then picks up the waste gas, carbon dioxide, which is passed out in the lungs.

Anemia is a reduction in the number of red blood cells and/or in the quantity of hemoglobin. Anemia is not itself a disease, but a sign of disease in the blood or in another part of the body.

There are numerous causes of anemia, but for clarity they are broken down into three groups.

1. *Blood loss,* which can be acute or chronic, and is most commonly due to: hemorrhage (bleeding) from trauma, disease, or parasites and blood coagulation disorders such as hemophilia.

2. *Decreased red cell production* from: dietary deficiencies, such as lack of iron, copper, some of the B vitamins, vitamin E, and poor or low-protein diets; parasites, external or internal; infections; kidney or liver failure; cancer; destruction of bone marrow (aplastic anemia) from radiation, drugs, infections, and poisons.

3. *Increased red cell destruction* from hemolytic anemias, in which the red blood cells are destroyed in the circulation. The causes include: congenital defects, parasites, abnormalities of the immune system, and cancer.

SYMPTOMS Acute blood loss leads to weakness, a rapid pulse, increased heart and respiratory rate, collapse, and shock.

Chronic blood-loss signs are less obvious. The dog tires readily, is lethargic and weak, has pale gums, and an increased heart and respiratory rate.

DIAGNOSIS The diagnosis is made by the history, the symptoms, and a physical examination, and is confirmed by blood tests. Microscopic examination of the blood cells can lead to a specific diagnosis in many anemias.

TREATMENT Acute blood loss is an emergency situation and requires immediate treatment to stop the bleeding which, particularly in trauma cases, may require surgery. Dogs, like people, have a number of different blood groups and need to have blood typed and matched before repeated transfusions. Treatment for shock will be necessary if the blood loss is severe (*see* Chapter 16, Emergency Care; Emergency Cases: Shock). Blood transfusions, intravenous fluids, and blood replacement products will also be necessary.

Chronic blood loss is not an emergency situation, and treatment should be directed at eliminating the cause. Unless the dog is very anemic, most anemias can be treated by high-protein diets, iron, and vitamin supplements, particularly if the primary cause can be identified and he responds to treatment.

9

The Reproductive System

We will discuss the reproductive systems of the male and female dog separately.

MALE GENITAL SYSTEM DISEASES AND DISORDERS

Diseases and disorders of the male genital system will be discussed under the individual organs that are most often affected.

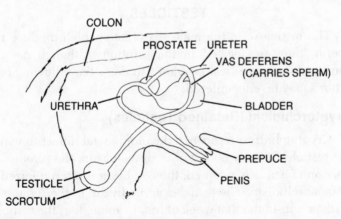

Male Reproductive and Urinary Systems

PENIS

The penis is the male genitalia.

Balanoposthitis (Inflammation of the Penis)

Balanoposthitis is an inflammation of the penis. The most common causes are the presence of foreign bodies such as grass awns; trauma from accidents; and bacterial infections.

SYMPTOMS Pus is usually seen discharging from the prepuce (foreskin), the penis is irritated and swollen, and the dog licks the area.

DIAGNOSIS Diagnosis is made from the symptoms and a physical examination. Laboratory tests and a culture and sensitivity test on the discharge may be required in some cases.

TREATMENT Treatment involves flushing the prepuce with an antiseptic, removal of any foreign body, and the use of antibiotics locally and sometimes also by mouth if a bacterial infection is involved. Most cases respond well to treatment.

Sometimes a pus discharge from the prepuce is coming from disease in other male genital organs or the urinary tract, and in these instances investigation and treatment of the primary cause will be necessary.

TESTICLES

The testicles are the male sex organs which produce the sperm; they are located in the scrotum. Although not the source of many medical problems in dogs, the following conditions may be encountered:

Cryptorchidism (Retained Testicles)

Cryptorchidism refers to a developmental defect in which the testicles, one or both, fail to descend into the scrotum. If only one testicle is retained, the condition is often referred to as monorchidism. The testicles normally are in the scrotum at birth or within the first week of life. In some dogs the testicles do not descend until puberty, at about seven months of age.

TREATMENT There is no treatment to correct this condition; male hormones have been used but are seldom effective. Affected purebred dogs may not be shown and should not be bred as the condition can be hereditary. Retained testicles have a higher incidence of tumors, and for this reason castration to remove the retained testicle(s) is often recommended.

Orchitis

Orchitis is an inflammation of the testicle. The causes are trauma, infection, or rotation of the testicle.

SYMPTOMS The affected testicle will feel hot and swollen, and will be painful; loss of appetite and fever may accompany the orchitis.

DIAGNOSIS Diagnosis is made from the symptoms and a physical examination.

TREATMENT If the testicle is twisted, surgical correction may be required. Abscesses must be drained. Most cases of orchitis respond to antibiotics, tranquilizers, pain killers, and the use of hot packs. If the orchitis is secondary to a prostate disease, the primary disease must also be treated.

PROSTATE GLAND

The prostate gland is located at the neck of the bladder and secretes a milky fluid, which bathes the sperm. A number of problems involve this gland in the dog.

Prostatitis

Prostatitis is an inflammation of the prostate gland. Most infections arise in the urinary tract or are carried via the blood from an infection site in another area of the body.

SYMPTOMS The condition is painful, and there is loss of appetite, fever, and vomiting; the dog will move reluctantly and with the back arched.

DIAGNOSIS The veterinarian diagnoses this condition from the history, clinical signs, and a physical examination that will include palpation of the gland via the rectum. Laboratory tests on washings from the urethra and a urine sample will confirm the diagnosis. X-rays may be required in some cases.

TREATMENT Treatment with antibiotics is effective in most cases, although a culture and sensitivity test may be required to determine which antibiotic to use. If abscessed, surgical drainage may be necessary. Some cases become chronic and are complicated by chronic cystitis.

Prostatic Hyperplasia (Enlarged Prostate)

Most unaltered male dogs over five years of age have some prostatic hyperplasia, which is an increase in size of the prostate gland. (This is also a common problem in older men.) In dogs, the condition is thought to be related to a hormonal imbalance.

SYMPTOMS If the gland becomes very enlarged there may be difficulty in urinating, straining to urinate, and dribbling of urine. Otherwise, the condition appears to be painless.

DIAGNOSIS The veterinarian can diagnose the condition by palpating the gland via the rectum. A biopsy may be recommended to rule out a tumor as the cause of the enlargement.

TREATMENT Castration is the best treatment and results in permanent reduction in size of the gland. For dog owners who do not want to have the dog castrated, administration of female hormones will often effectively reduce the size of the gland. However, there are hazardous side effects if the dog has to be kept on them on a long-term basis.

Tumors

The testicles and prostate are quite frequently the sites of both benign and malignant tumors. (*See* Chapter 15, Cancer; *and* Chapter 4, The Skin; Hormonal Skin Diseases: Male Dogs—Sex Hormone Problems, for further information.)

FEMALE GENITAL SYSTEM DISEASES AND DISORDERS

The female genital system is much more complicated than the male system, and as a result medical problems are encountered relatively frequently in the unspayed (or "intact") female dog. They are discussed under the individual organs.

OVARIES

The ovaries are the female sex organs which produce the ova (eggs); they are located in the abdominal cavity behind the kidneys. The two main diseases which affect the ovaries in the dog are cysts und tumors.

Ovarian Cysts

The exact cause of ovarian cysts cannot always be determined, but hormone imbalances are involved. Cysts of the ovary usually produce excessive quantities of estrogen.

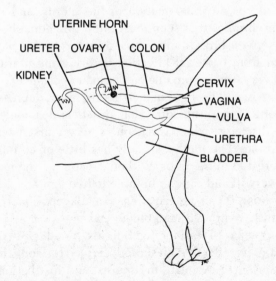

Female Reproductive and Urinary Systems

SYMPTOMS A dog with ovarian cysts is nervous, irritable, has a swollen vulva, and is attractive to males and may mate, but is usually sterile.

TREATMENT The recommended treatment is an ovariohysterectomy (spay), which completely resolves all symptoms.

Ovarian Tumors

Unfortunately, ovarian tumors in the dog are usually large and have spread before signs are seen. Surgery is the treatment of choice, but the prognosis is poor in most cases. (*See* Chapter 15, Cancer.)

UTERUS

Uterine disease is not a common problem in veterinary medicine, because so many female dogs are spayed today. However, in the unspayed female dog, the following uterine diseases are quite frequently encountered.

Metritis

Metritis is an inflammation of the uterus, and it can be acute or chronic. It is seen most often immediately after the dog has given birth, and is caused by a retained placenta or fetus, or from bacterial infection entering the uterus during the delivery (often from unclean human assistance).

SYMPTOMS The signs of metritis are fever, depression, loss of appetite, vomiting, diarrhea, thirst, and a foul-smelling uterine discharge which is red and watery at first, later becoming pustular. The mother usually has little or no milk and is not interested in the pups. Without treatment, the mother becomes very ill and can die in three to five days.

DIAGNOSIS The veterinarian can diagnose metritis from the history, symptoms, and blood tests.

TREATMENT Treatment with fluids, blood tranfusions, and antibiotics is effective if started early. Hormone injections may be used to evacuate the uterus, and instillation of antibiotics into the uterus is used in some cases.

In some dogs, metritis becomes a chronic disease. Although the dog looks relatively healthy, there is a low-grade uterine infection, and she may fail to conceive, or if she does conceive, the pups are often born dead or die within a few days of birth. Antibiotics are used to treat chronic metritis, but are not always successful in curing the disease. Unless the dog is very valuable for breeding, spaying is recommended in these cases.

Pyometra

Pyometra refers to a pus-filled uterus. The condition is seen most often in unspayed female dogs over five years old and is caused by an ovarian dysfunction in which too much of the female sex hormone progesterone is produced.

SYMPTOMS Initially, the dog appears healthy, although the abdomen can be swollen from the enlarged uterus, and a watery-to-pus-like uterine discharge may be seen. As the disease progresses, the dog becomes depressed and has loss of appetite, vomiting, fever, or a subnormal temperature; the vulva may be swollen. Many dogs go on for months without the disease worsening. However, if the cervix (neck of the uterus) closes and there is no further discharge, acute and serious illness often occurs, which may be accompanied by signs of kidney failure.

DIAGNOSIS Veterinary diagnosis is made by the history, clinical signs, palpation of the enlarged uterus, blood tests, and in some cases, x-rays.

TREATMENT The treatment is surgical removal of the uterus and ovaries. If the dog is seriously ill, she will need extensive supportive medical care to survive the surgery. For this reason, early treatment of this disease is recommended.

MAMMARY GLANDS

Inflammation and tumors of the mammary glands are not uncommon in the unspayed female dog. These diseases are almost never seen in spayed females.

Mastitis

Mastitis is an inflammation of the mammary glands. It is seen most frequently following birth, or occasionally from wounds or bruises to this area. Infection from bacteria can also occur.

Symptoms

The glands are hot, swollen, painful, and a purple color, especially if infected. The dog will often have a fever, poor appetite, and be depressed. A watery to bloody or pus-like discharge may be seen at the teat; sometimes the gland becomes abscessed and ruptures, with tissue breakdown and a heavy pus discharge.

DIAGNOSIS Diagnosis is made from the symptoms and a physical examination. Culture and sensitivity testing on the discharges may be required. Other laboratory tests may be necessary if the dog is very ill.

TREATMENT Treatment involves the use of antibiotics, hot packs on the affected glands, and removal of the pups. If an abscess is present, it may have to be surgically drained. Drugs may also have to be given to stop the milk production. Most cases respond well to treatment, although the glands can become chronically scarred if the infection is extensive.

Tumors

Mammary tumors are the most common neoplasms (cancers) in unspayed female dogs. (*See* Chapter 15, Cancer.)

VAGINA AND VULVA

Infections of the vulva or vagina are usually accompanied by a discharge and swelling of the tissues in the affected area. The causative agents are bacteria, and most cases respond well to antibiotic ointments locally; in severe infections, antibiotics may be given by injection or orally as well. Chronic cases may require further diagnostic work.

REPRODUCTION

Estrus Cycle (Heat)

A female dog reaches puberty between six and ten months of age. She normally has two estrus (heat) cycles a year, each cycle lasting about three weeks. There are four stages in the estrus cycle:

1. *Anestrus.* This is the quiescent period of the cycle from the end of estrus to the beginning of proestrus, and it lasts about three months.

2. *Proestrus.* During this period there is swelling of the vulva and a watery, red discharge can be observed. It lasts seven to nine days and the female will not accept a male during this period.

3. *Estrus.* The vulva area becomes even more swollen and the discharge becomes paler in color. It lasts about nine days, and during this period the female ovulates and accepts the male.

4. *Metestrus.* This is the stage of regression of all the signs of estrus and it lasts about two months, although the discharge ceases in about one week. After this stage the dog enters the inactive period of anestrus.

The veterinarian can determine which stage of an estrus cycle a dog is in by examining smears of the vaginal discharges microscopically. These tests can be very helpful in determining the best period to mate the female to the male to ensure a successful breeding, and are used particularly for dogs which refuse to mate or cannot be brought to the male because of distance limitations, and have to be bred by artificial insemination.

False Pregnancy

Following the heat period, some females—particularly those which are older or have been bred and not become pregnant—will go through what is called a false pregnancy. This can last from one to three months, during which time the abdomen appears swollen, there may be a slight vulvar discharge, and the mammary glands swell and sometimes even produce milk. Some of these dogs make a nest and appear to go through labor.

This condition is thought to be caused by a hormone imbalance. Although most cases do not require treatment, it can be treated with hormones if the signs are severe. A dog which exhibits false pregnancy will continue to do so after each heat period, and spaying is recommended unless the dog is being used for breeding.

Mating

Dogs seldom need any assistance with mating, since it is an instinctive process. When the female is ready to accept the male, she will allow the male to mount and enter her. Once the male has penetrated her, the penis swells and the dogs become what is referred to as "locked" or "tied." This can last as long as thirty minutes and attempts should never be made to separate them or damage to the penis and vagina may occur. Separating them at this point will not prevent pregnancy since the male ejaculates just after penetration; thus sperm are already present in the vagina.

Females will mate a number of times during the receptive period and with many different males, if available. As a result fertilization of separate ova by sperm cells of different males during the same heat is possible. This is called superfecundation, and explains why puppies of many different breed-types of dogs can be born to the same mother at the same time.

Pregnancy

Few healthy dogs need much care during pregnancy, although all should have had a veterinary examination prior to mating and have been vaccinated and wormed. The normal gestation period in dogs is from fifty-eight to sixty-five days.

Abdominal swelling will be noticeable after about five weeks and your veterinarian can usually palpate the fetuses in the abdomen as early as three to four weeks. The mammary glands will also enlarge, and this is particularly noticeable in the first pregnancy. Sometimes, depending on the breed of dog, the veterinarian can even make an educated guess on how many puppies are developing, although it becomes more difficult to palpate the fetuses individually as the pregnancy progresses. At about forty-five days, the fetal skeletons can be seen on an x-ray.

During the last three weeks of pregnancy, extra food, more frequent feedings, and a vitamin and mineral supplement are sometimes recommended.

Abortions and miscarriages do occur in dogs if bacterial infections such as brucellosis occur or if other uterine problems or infections are present (*see* Female Genital System Diseases and Disorders, earlier in this chapter).

Whelping or Delivery (Parturition)

There are three stages of labor:

First stage. During the early onset stages of labor, the dog will become restless, anxious, refuse food, and sometimes pant. The body temperature will drop to as low as 98° Fahrenheit, and there may be a watery vaginal discharge and milk coming from the nipples. She will seek an area to whelp, preferably a whelping box which has been prepared, and will settle down here. This first stage lasts from twelve to twenty-four hours normally.

Second stage. Uterine contractions and straining can be seen as the abdominal muscles contract in her effort to expel the puppies. Most puppies are born at fifteen- to sixty-minute intervals, although this is very variable and sometimes two puppies are born close together. On the average all puppies are born in about six hours, but it can take as long as twenty hours.

Third stage. This is the uterine resting stage and occurs

between each birth. It usually lasts about fifteen minutes, sometimes up to an hour. The mother tends to the puppies which have been born at this stage and may even walk around and take a drink of water.

Preferably the dog should be left alone during labor; the fewer interruptions and spectators, the better. Some nervous dogs may stop labor altogether if disturbed or moved. The best thing is quietly to check her and the puppies already born periodically to be sure there are no problems, keeping in mind that many whelping problems and uterine infections are caused by too much well-intentioned human interference.

Difficult Birth (Dystocia)

First, it should be mentioned that posterior (breech) presentation is normal in dogs, and occurs in up to 40% of deliveries. Recognizing birthing difficulties and at what point emergency veterinary care is needed can be a problem for the inexperienced dog breeder. The signs that the mother or pups are in trouble are:

1. A pup is seen at the external birth canal and is not expelled in a few minutes.

2. The mother is in obvious labor (straining) for over two hours and no pup is delivered. This must not be confused with the resting stage between births which can extend up to four hours, but there will be no straining then.

3. There is excessive bleeding.

4. The mother is obviously in distress.

5. The mother does not break the sac the pup is usually born in, clean off the pup, or bite the umbilical cord.

6. No placenta (afterbirth) is expelled after a pup is born. This is not always easy to determine as the mother frequently eats the afterbirth.

If the mother cannot deliver the pups, veterinary care will involve the use of hormone injections to assist labor, or the puppies will have to be delivered by caesarean section if contractions do not occur or if there is an obstruction to delivery. It is advisable to spay the mother at the same time, as she will probably have similar problems with further pregnancies.

If the mother ignores the puppy at birth, it will be necessary to break the sac, wrap the puppy in a towel and rub it vigorously, swing the head down to drain the fluid from the lungs, and wipe the fluid out of the mouth, all of which should help the puppy start breathing. If this is not successful, blowing into the mouth may stimulate breathing. The pup should then be returned to the mother.

Most mothers go through pregnancy and delivery without any problems, but it is a good idea to have a new mother and the puppies examined by the veterinarian within a few days of birth, particularly if you suspect the mother is unwell or the puppies are not thriving. A greenish uterine discharge, which changes to brownish and then to clear mucus will be present for up to three weeks after birth. If this discharge is bloody, pus-like, or foul smelling, there is probably a retained fetus, placenta, or uterine infection, and veterinary care is essential to save the mother and the pups.

If no problems arise the mother dog will take care of herself and her puppies without any assistance—except that she will require up to three times the normal amount of food, and if the litter is large, a good vitamin and mineral supplement will be helpful.

Eclampsia (Milk Fever)

This is a condition that may occur a few weeks after delivery, caused by too low blood calcium levels. It requires immediate emergency treatment (*see* Chapter 16, Emergency Care; Emergency Cases: Eclampsia).

Puppy Care

There are many excellent publications available on puppy care, and anyone planning on breeding a dog should become well informed in this area. Fortunately, the mother does most of the work of caring for the puppies for the first six weeks of life. The eyes open at about two weeks of age. The puppies should be encouraged to start eating at about three weeks of age to relieve the nutritional drain on the mother. Weaning should start about five weeks of age, and all puppies should be fully weaned by eight weeks of age. If milk production does not stop naturally, remove the mother from the pups, stop all food and water for twenty-four hours, and then reduce the food to the normal before-pregnancy amount. Between six and eight weeks of age, the puppies (and a stool sample) should be brought to the veterinarian so they can be checked for worms and have a physical check-up, and to make arrangements for the start of a vaccination schedule.

Orphan Puppies

Caring for orphan puppies is a time-consuming job, and despite the best care, it is not always easy to save their lives. They need to be kept warm (over 85° Fahrenheit the first week); fed six or more times a day with special formulas available from veterinarians or pet stores, using baby bottles or eye droppers; massaged after each feeding with a warm cotton swab in the genital and anal areas to stimulate urination and defecation; and not handled too much in between these ministrations. If they make it through the first few weeks, most will survive, although these puppies often have psychological problems in relating to other dogs when they mature.

BIRTH CONTROL

Recent figures from the United States Department of Agriculture make us realize what a deplorable situation the pet overpopulation problem is, particularly in a country which so values life, both animal and human. About 20 million dogs and cats a year are no longer wanted. Of these, an estimated 5 million are abandoned and presumably die from starvation, disease, or accidents. Only 2 million of those brought to pounds or shelters are returned to their owners or adopted; the remaining 13 million are destroyed. In round figures, this works out to one-quarter of a million every week; 36,000 every day; 1,500 every hour; 25 every minute; or one every two seconds. These figures are higher if the abandoned animals are included. With statistics like these, it is obvious that birth control for pets is most important. The following methods of birth control are available for dogs:

NEUTERING, OR ALTERING

The terms neutering or altering are used by the public when referring to an animal in which the reproductive organs have been removed surgically. In the female the surgery is called an ovariohysterectomy or a spay, and in the male it is called an orchiectomy or a castration. These surgeries are still the most satisfactory methods of birth control for dogs, although continuing research is being conducted to develop alternative, less hazardous, and less costly methods.

Spay (Ovariohysterectomy)

The word "spay" originates from the Middle French verb *espeer*, meaning to cut with a sword. In late Middle English, it meant to operate upon a female to remove the ovaries and destroy the reproductive power. In veterinary medicine today it means the ovariohysterectomy, the removal of both the ovaries and the uterus. The dog is then said to be spayed.

Spaying is major abdominal surgery done under full anesthesia; however, because veterinarians perform this surgery so frequently, fatalities are rare. A female dog should be spayed before her first heat, but not earlier than five to six months of age. At that point, the surgery is less complicated, less risky, and as a result, less costly. Many dog owners believe that a dog should go through one heat period or have one pregnancy before spaying, but there is no justification for this, although this rumor refuses to die! If a female dog is allowed to go through her first heat, she will develop more fully in the physical sense (called "fixing the breed characteristics"), but the average dog owner would not be aware of these fine points, and once a purebred dog has been spayed, she cannot be used for showing or breeding anyway. Also, the surgery is more difficult, and therefore more hazardous and costly, following the first heat or a pregnancy.

The advantages of spaying are many:

1. The dog cannot become pregnant.
2. The dog owner is not contributing to the dog overpopulation problem.
3. There are no more periods of heat, during which the female will be restless and have to be confined, and the nuisance factor of male dogs hanging around your home and fighting will also be eliminated.
4. The dangers of uterine and ovarian infections and cancer are eliminated.
5. Cancer of the mammary glands (breast), the leading cancer in unspayed female dogs, is extremely rare in spayed females.
6. The spayed female dog is more devoted to the owner, because she is not distracted by mating, pregnancy, and caring for puppies.
7. On the average, spayed females live longer than unspayed females and are healthier.

There are also disadvantages to spaying, including:

1. The risk of surgery. However, fatalities are very rare, particularly if done when the dog is young and healthy.
2. Spayed females may become fat and lazy. It is true that estrogen, the hormone produced by the ovaries, inhibits food intake and weight gain, but since this hormone is only present at a high level in the unspayed female dog for a few weeks,

twice a year, this is not a significant factor in keeping un-spayed females slim. Other facts are that spayed females do have somewhat reduced physical activity, and do not have the additional burdens on the body of pregnancy and lactation. If all these facts are taken into account, it is obvious that if a spayed female does become fat and lazy, it is because the owner is overfeeding and underexercising the dog.

3. Some older spayed female dogs dribble urine and have loss of hair because of low production of estrogen. This is by no means a common problem and is readily treated with hormone replacement drugs (*see* Chapter 4, The Skin; Hormonal Skin Diseases: Female Dogs—Sex Hormone Problems, Hypoestrogenism, for further information).

Surgical Alternatives to Spaying

Many dog owners ask veterinarians why the tubes are not tied, as is frequently done as a method of birth control in women. There is really no advantage in tying off the fallopian tubes in dogs, as they will continue to come into heat and mate, and these nuisance factors will not be eliminated.

Other alternative surgeries are to remove just the ovaries or the uterus. It has been found that if only the ovaries are removed, there is an increased risk of later uterine infections, which then entails additional surgery, risk, and expense for the dog owner. Removing only the uterus has the same disadvantages as tying the tubes—the dog continues to come into heat.

Castration (Orchiectomy)

Castration has not been used in dogs as a method of pet population control to any great extent, but it is being done more frequently now, as many humane societies and animal shelters have made it mandatory before they will allow a male dog to be adopted. Castration is the removal of the testicles and following this operation, the male hormone (testosterone) level is reduced. Many castrated dogs will still attempt to mate, but are no longer fertile and cannot impregnate the female.

As in spaying, the advantages of castration are many:

1. The dog owner is not contributing to the dog overpopulation problem.

2. The danger of testicle infections and cancer are eliminated.

3. Prostate gland enlargements and infections are seldom seen in castrated dogs.

4. Castrated dogs roam or break out of their home premises less and are therefore not as likely to be injured in accidents.

5. Objectional sexual behavior is reduced or eliminated.

6. Aggressiveness is also reduced. However, this will not make a dog less aggressive protecting its owner or home, but rather, less likely to fight with other dogs over females.

7. Dogs that tend to urinate in the house will often stop this behavior following castration.

8. Castrated dogs are more devoted to the owner and more content to stay home, because they are not hormonally driven to seek out females in heat continually.

9. Castrated dogs live longer on the average than intact males and are healthier.

Again, there are disadvantages to castration, including:

1. The risk of surgery. However, castration is not major surgery, and the only serious risk is from the anesthetic, which almost never leads to a complication in a young, healthy dog.

2. The castrated dog appears less masculine as the muscles are softer and less well developed.

3. Although they persist, the fat-and-lazy and less-joy-in-living labels are myths. On the contrary, castration results in reduced food intake and loss of weight in dogs, and the only change in the dog's behavior is that it is more attached to the owner and less interested in other dogs and in roaming.

As a method of birth control, castration, of course, is not nearly as effective as spaying the female, because one intact male in a neighborhood can impregnate all the females without any problem!

Surgical Alternatives to Castration

Many dog owners, particularly male owners, object to castrating their dogs, for obvious macho reasons. If they are seriously concerned about the pet population problem, an alternative is to have the dog vasectomized, which involves the removal of a piece of the tubes that carry the sperm. This will leave the dog fully masculine, but will make it sterile.

BIRTH CONTROL PILLS

Oral birth control pills are available and approved for use in female dogs. Like their human counterparts, they are not without hazard and should only be used for planned parenthood for breeding female dogs or for dog owners who object to neutering on principle.

There are two such drugs available at present:

Megestrol Acetate

Megestrol acetate is designed to postpone estrus (heat) in dogs. The dosage and number of days of treatment (eight to thirty-two days) depend on what stage of the estrus cycle the dog is in when the drug is started. The drug is available in tablet form and can be given by mouth or crushed and mixed in the food. Side effects are minor and temporary, and include increased appetite, decreased activity, weight gain, and, rarely, mammary enlargement with lactation.

The manufacturers recommend that megestrol acetate should not be used in dogs with uterine disease, prior to or during the first estrus cycle, in pregnant dogs, or in dogs with mammary tumors; nor should it be used for more than two consecutive treatments.

Following treatment, estrus is postponed on the average four to six months.

Mibolerone

Mibolerone can be used for long periods of estrus prevention and is available in liquid form. It requires a daily dosage by mouth or added to the food. It must be started between estrus cycles to be effective. This drug must be used only in healthy, mature, nonlactating dogs.

Few side effects are seen, except if given to dogs younger than seven months; these will show signs of masculinization, so such use is not recommended even if the dog appears to be mature at this age. The manufacturers recommend discontinuing this drug after twenty-four months of use.

There is continuing research on birth control medications for dogs, both for the male and the female. No doubt safer and more effective products will be developed.

CONFINEMENT

This is an obvious method of birth control, but it is not as easy as it sounds, particularly for the female dog. When in heat, usually twice yearly, she will have to be confined for as long as three weeks. During part of this period she will attempt to escape, and the males will make every effort to get to her, which will cause a considerable nuisance, not to mention property damage. Most dog owners are not prepared to put up with this, and despite very careful confinement, a surprising number of females still manage to become pregnant! There are products available to reduce the male attractant odor of the female in heat, but they are only partially effective.

ABORTION

Abortion is seldom used as a method of birth control in dogs. The main reason is that in most instances when a dog owner requests an abortion, the dog is already too advanced in the pregnancy for abortion. The only alternative at this point is either a caesarean or a spay.

MISMATING

If a female dog is accidentally bred, a pregnancy can be prevented with the use of estrogen hormones, by injection or by mouth. The earlier these drugs are administered following the mating, the more successful the results. Unfortunately, these hormones will make the female attractive to males, and she may continue mating, although she will not usually become pregnant. These drugs have other undesirable side effects and should not be used routinely as a birth control method in dogs.

INTRAUTERINE AND INTRAVAGINAL DEVICES

Both these devices have been tried in female dogs, but neither has been entirely successful to date.

BREEDING

Dog Breeding Is Not for Everyone

Many dog owners after they have purchased an expensive purebred female think it would be fun to breed her, and all too often the motive is to make money and recoup the cost of the purchase. No veterinarian encourages this type of breeding—not for moralistic reasons, but because the scenario goes something like this:

First dog owners will have to study the bloodlines of the breed, obtain expert advice (for which they may have to pay) and then take the time and trouble to seek out the right male to breed their female to (a service for which a fee will be charged). Prior to the breeding, the female should be examined by a veterinarian, vaccinated, and wormed—all additional expenses. Even if the breeding and pregnancy go smoothly, the average pet owner invariably runs into problems with the delivery. Many times, these delivery problems are not real, but result from a lack of experience on the part of the owner. The first-time or amateur breeder either rushes to the veterinarian at the first signs of labor, or fails to recognize when the dog is having serious problems and does not seek veterinary help in time to save the pups and the mother. Either way, this lack of experience costs money.

Even if all goes smoothly and the dog produces a nice litter of puppies, the chances of further problems and complications increase from this point on. For instance, the dog may not be an adequate mother. She may neglect her puppies or even kill them, have no milk, have a postdelivery infection, or the puppies may be weak or get sick, just to name a few of the problems that can arise. If 50% of the litter survive, the owner will have done well.

Now, the puppies have to be cared for, weaned, fed, cleaned, vaccinated, and wormed, all time-consuming jobs and additional veterinary expense. The puppies then have to be advertised for sale, and registration papers have to be obtained in order to ask purebred prices. At this point the owner runs into the realities of the dog breeding business, which is that the pet-buying public generally does not want to spend much money and is unaware of the cost of breeding, while the customers most likely to seek out a purebred are often knowledgeable to the point of being able to undermine the owner's confidence in the prices asked. If the puppies are not sold by ten weeks of age, it may be hard even to give them away.

It is most often the experience of amateur breeders that when they add up their out-of-pocket expenses and deduct the money received from sales (if any), the result will be negative, without even counting the labor they have invested. It is at this point the veterinarian receives a call from such an owner requesting an immediate spay and giving the long, sad story of the happy breeding experience that went awry, which the experienced and sensible veterinarian advised against in the first place!

If, despite all this, dog owners want to breed their dogs, they should purchase a good book on breeding dogs and another on general dog care. A veterinarian can also provide information and free literature on these subjects.

CONGENITAL DEFECTS IN DOGS

Congenital defects are abnormalities of body structure or function present at birth. Most are caused by an inherited genetic defect; some are due to damage to the fetus during development. Inherited or genetically caused congenital defects run in families and some of the most frequently encountered in dogs are listed in the following chart:

Congenital Defects in Dogs

Congenital Defect*	Breeds Most Commonly Affected
EYES	
Cataracts	German shepherd, golden retriever, bull terrier, Labrador retriever, beagle, standard poodle, miniature schnauzer, Boston terrior.
Ectropion	Many breeds.
Entropion	Many breeds.

Congenital Defects in Dogs *(continued)*

Congenital Defect*	Breeds Most Commonly Affected
Distichiasis	Pekingese, poodle, cocker spaniel, Irish setter, English bulldog, golden retriever, Saint Bernard.
Trichiasis	Pug, Pekingese.
Retinal Atrophy	Labrador retriever, golden retriever, English springer and cocker spaniels, border collie, Irish setter, miniature and toy poodle, Norwegian elkhound, Welsh corgi.

EARS

Deafness	Bull terrier. Often associated with white coat color in Dalmatian, collie, and fox terrier.

NERVOUS SYSTEM

Abnormal Behavior	Several breeds.
Epilepsy	German shepherd, keeshond, collie, beagle.
Hydrocephalus	Chihuahua, cocker spaniel, English bulldog.

URINARY SYSTEM

Cystine Calculi	Irish terrier, dachshund, Labrador retriever, miniature poodle, boxer, German shepherd, Welsh corgi, great Dane, Scottish terrier.
Urate Calculi	Dalmatian.

REPRODUCTIVE SYSTEM

Cryptorchidism	Most breeds.
Dystocia	English bulldog, Welsh corgi, greyhound, most miniature breeds.
Uterine Inertia	Border, Aberdeen, and Scottish terriers.

BLOOD SYSTEM

Hemophilia and Other Bleeding Disorders	Many breeds.

CARDIOVASCULAR SYSTEM

Heart Defects	Boxer, miniature and toy poodle, German shepherd, Irish setter, great Dane, Newfoundland, English bulldog, Chihuahua, collie, Pomeranian, cocker spaniel, beagle.

RESPIRATORY SYSTEM

Trachea Collapse	Toy and miniature breeds.

Congenital Defects in Dogs *(continued)*

Congenital Defect*	Breeds Most Commonly Affected
Narrow Nostrils and Long Soft Palate	Bulldog, Boston terrier.
Esophageal Dilation	Many breeds.

ENDOCRINE SYSTEM

Diabetes Mellitus	Dachshund, Samoyed, King Charles spaniel.
Dwarfism	German shepherd.

SKELETAL SYSTEM

Cleft Lip and Palate	English bulldog, Shih Tzu, dachshund, cocker spaniel, German shepherd, beagle.
Extra Teeth	Boxer, English bulldog.
Hemivertebra	English bulldog, Boston terrier, and many small and screw tail breeds.
Intervertebral Disc Disease	Dachshund, Pekingese, cocker spaniel, beagle.
Spina Bifida	English bulldog.
Elbow Dysplasia	Many large and giant breeds.
Hip Dysplasia	Mostly large and giant breeds. Also in cocker spaniel and Shetland sheepdog.
Epiphyseal Dysplasia	Beagle.
Patellar Luxation	Pomeranian, Yorkshire terrier, Chihuahua, Boston terrier, miniature and toy poodle.

MUSCULAR SYSTEM

Inguinal Hernia	Basset hound, basenji, Pekingese, Lhasa Apso.
Umbilical Hernia	Collie, cocker spaniel, bull terrier, basenji, Airedale terrier, Pekingese, pointer, Weimaraner.

IMMUNE SYSTEM

Demodectic Mange	Several breeds.
Nasal Solar Dermatitis	Collie, Shetland sheepdog.

* See specific disease for detailed description.

10

The Digestive System

The function of the digestive system is to ingest food and water, break down the food, absorb the nutrients into the bloodstream, and eliminate the waste materials. The digestive

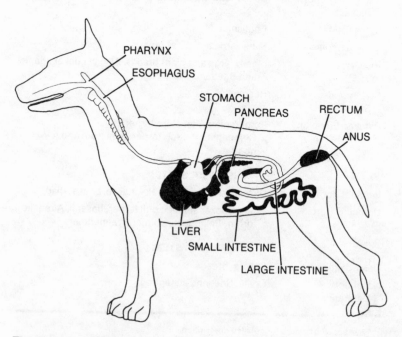

The Digestive System

system starts at the mouth, and from there passes on into the pharynx, esophagus, stomach, small intestines, large intestines, rectum, and anus. It also includes other organs, such as the pancreas and liver, which produce enymes used in the digestive processes.

Many medical problems occur in the digestive system of the dog, but emphasis here will be on those most frequently encountered, and therefore, of most concern to the dog owner.

DIAGNOSIS OF DIGESTIVE SYSTEM DISEASES AND DISORDERS

Diagnosing the cause of digestive system disorders in dogs can be difficult, and depending on the severity of the problem, will require some or all of the folowing approaches:

1. *History.* The dog's medical history can be most helpful to the veterinarian in making a diagnosis in digestive system disorders. Give the veterinarian a detailed description of the dog's symptoms, appetite, and diet, the length of the illness, and previous medical history.

2. *Physical examination.* Your veterinarian will need to examine the dog. Disorders in the mouth and throat may be readily visible, and abnormalities of the stomach, liver, or intestinal tract may be found by palpating the abdomen.

3. *X-rays.* X-ray examination is often necessary to reach a diagnosis; this type of examination may require administering a contrast material, such as barium, by mouth or by rectum. The barium coats the intestinal tract and makes defects more visible on the x-rays.

4. *Laboratory tests.* There are many laboratory tests available for diagnosing digestive problems in dogs. These include: tests on the feces to identify parasites, infectious agents, poor absorption of food, and bleeding in the gastrointestinal tract; blood and urine tests; and tests which measure

liver, kidney, and pancreatic function. Culture and sensitivity testing may be required in bacterial infections.

5. *Biopsies.* Microscopic examination of tissue samples may be necessary to diagnose some digestive diseases or to identify tumors.

6. *Exploratory surgery.* Some digestive diseases and disorders cannot be diagnosed by any of the previous procedures, and exploratory surgery of the abdominal cavity may be the only means of reaching a diagnosis.

MOUTH DISEASES AND DISORDERS

Cheilitis (Lip Inflammation)

Cheilitis is an inflammation affecting the lips; it can be caused by injury, by irritation or from excessive tartar, or, in some breeds of dogs, from infection in deep lip folds.

SYMPTOMS AND DIAGNOSIS The lesions can be observed and diagnosis can be made from the history and a physical examination.

TREATMENT Preferred treatment involves removal of the cause, cleaning and medicating the area involved, and sometimes the use of antibiotics and corticosteroids by injection or by mouth.

Stomatitis (Mouth Inflammation)

Stomatitis is an inflammation of the tissues lining the mouth, due, most commonly, to bacterial, fungal, or viral infections. Other causes are: niacin deficiency, injury from chemicals or poisons, dental disease, or an accompanying symptom to another systemic or immune system disease.

SYMPTOMS The signs of stomatitis include loss of appetite or reluctance to eat, excessive salivation or drooling, evidence of pain when the mouth is examined, and a foul mouth odor.

DIAGNOSIS The diagnosis can be made by examination of the mouth. The affected areas will be reddened and ulcerated. A microscopic examination of the mouth discharges can be diagnostic.

TREATMENT Treatment involves removal of the cause if possible, cleaning of the lesions, and administration of pain killers if necessary. Doses of antibiotics, corticosteroids, and atropine to reduce the excessive salivation may be required in some cases. A soft diet or even force-feeding may be recommended for a few days or until there is a response to treatment.

Oral Papillomatosis (Warts)

This is a contagious viral disease which occurs in young dogs.

SYMPTOMS Multiple warts, similar to human warts, occur in the mouth and pharynx, and on the tongue and lips. The skin around the mouth and other parts of the body is sometimes involved.

DIAGNOSIS The appearance and location of the warts are diagnostic.

TREATMENT The disease is self-limiting and the warts usually disappear in one to three months as the dog develops immunity to the virus that causes them. Surgical removal may be required if they are extensive and are interfering with eating or breathing. There is also a vaccine available, and a number of drugs have been used with success in reducing the size of the warts.

Gum and Tooth Disease (*See* Chapter 7, The Teeth.)

PHARYNGEAL DISEASES AND DISORDERS

Pharyngitis (Pharynx Inflammation)

The pharynx is the area between the mouth and the esophagus. Pharyngitis is an inflammation of the pharynx, and usually arises from the spread of bacterial infection caused by streptococcal or staphylococcal organisms from the mouth or nose. It can also be due to the presence of foreign bodies or occur secondarily to other infectious diseases.

SYMPTOMS The symptoms are loss of appetite, gagging and spitting up white foam, vomiting, coughing, and sometimes fever.

DIAGNOSIS Diagnosis is based on the history, symptoms, and an examination of the throat.

TREATMENT Most cases respond to treatment with antibiotics. Foreign bodies will need to be removed under anesthesia. A soft diet and/or force-feeding may also be necessary.

ESOPHAGEAL DISEASES AND DISORDERS

Esophagitis (Esophageal Inflammation)

The esophagus is the passage between the pharynx and the stomach. Esophagitis is an inflammation of the esophagus, and in dogs, the most common cause is irritation from foreign bodies such as bones. Other causes are chemicals and poisons, and a parasitic worm found in the southeast, called *Spirocerca lupi*, which burrows into the wall of the esophagus creating nodules that may eventually become cancerous.

SYMPTOMS Symptoms are loss of appetite, difficulty in swallowing, regurgitation of food, weight loss, and dehydration.

DIAGNOSIS Diagnosis is made from the history and a physical examination of the esophagus, requiring anesthesia and the use of an esophagoscope to view the inflamed area. Alternatively, a diagnosis can sometimes be made by x-ray.

TREATMENT Although some may require surgical removal, most foreign bodies can be removed with forceps which are used with an esophagoscope. There is no satisfactory treatment for the esophageal worm at present. Antibiotics, a soft diet, and/or force-feeding will be required in some cases.

Dilation of the Esophagus

This refers to a stretching of the esophagus, also called achalasia or megaesophagus. It is due to an abnormality of the nerves and muscles of the esophagus. Another cause is a congenital defect in the development of the blood vessels of the heart, called persistent right aortic arch, which constricts the esophagus, resulting in dilation.

SYMPTOMS Vomiting, particularly of solid food, is the most obvious sign. Puppies are affected more often, and loss of weight, failure to grow, and poor condition are evident as the disease progresses.

DIAGNOSIS The history, together with the clinical signs, is diagnostic, and can be confirmed by x-rays.

TREATMENT Some puppies outgrow the problem, but most do not. Feeding a soft, liquid-consistency diet from an elevated position, such as a step, may help swallowing. Antispasmodic drugs have been used in some instances. Depending on the cause of the dilation, surgery can be curative if it is done before the damage to the esophagus becomes irreversible.

STOMACH DISEASES AND DISORDERS

Vomiting

Vomiting in dogs is not unusual, but it is, nonetheless, abnormal. While vomiting by itself is not a disease, it is a sign of acute or chronic gastritis (irritation or inflammation of the stomach). The most common cause of vomiting in dogs is the eating of irritating substances, such as bones, grass, foreign objects, or spicy, decomposed, or contaminated foods. Overeating or exercising immediately following a meal can cause vomiting, particularly in puppies. More serious, but less common, causes of vomiting in dogs are severe food poisoning; parasites; poisons; intestinal obstruction; tumors of the gastrointestinal tract; shock; pancreatic disease; liver disease; kidney disease; infectious diseases, such as distemper, canine infectious hepatitis, and leptospirosis; pharyngitis and tonsillitis; diseases and disorders of the nervous system, and trauma.

SYMPTOMS Dogs having minor stomach upsets usually vomit the irritant substance; they may vomit frothy yellow fluid later, but otherwise do not appear distressed. Persistent or frequent vomiting, particularly if the vomitus is bile-stained or bloody and is accompanied by signs of weakness, pain, fever, and dehydration, is more serious and requires veterinary treatment.

DIAGNOSIS Diagnosis of the cause of vomiting can be difficult because the causes are so numerous. A detailed history, physical examination, laboratory tests, and x-rays may be of diagnostic value in cases of persistent vomiting.

TREATMENT

Home treatment. If a dog vomits once or twice, but otherwise appears healthy, professional treatment is not necessary; but some investigation into the source of the problem is desirable if this is a frequent or continuing problem.

Following a vomiting episode, withhold the dog's food for twenty-four hours and limit its water supply. For occasional mild vomiting, this procedure should take care of the problem.

If the vomiting episode has been severe, offer a small amount of bland food, such as baby food, rice, or boiled egg after the twenty-four hour restrictions, or use a homemade diet (*see* Chapter 1, Nutrition; Types of Diets for Dogs: Gastrointestinal Upset Diet), and continue to limit the water supply. Special diets, such as Prescription Diet i/d, from Hill's, are available from veterinarians. If no further vomiting occurs, repeat this feeding in six hours and then gradually over a few days return the dog to its normal diet. Antacids or protectants are useful but seldom necessary in cases of occasional vomiting. The human dosages given with these products should be adjusted for the dog's weight. These may be helpful provided they do not cause further vomiting when administered.

Vomiting caused by overeating or exercising immediately following a meal can be overcome by feeding smaller meals or feeding more frequently, and by restricting exercise after meals.

If this home-care treatment does not solve the problem or if the vomiting is persistent or increases in frequency, then veterinary treatment will be necessary.

Veterinary treatment. Be sure to bring a sample of the vomitus to the veterinary hospital, and give the veterinarian any information that may be helpful in reaching a diagnosis. Veterinary treatment approaches will vary, depending on the cause of the vomiting. Possible treatments may include:

1. Supportive and symptomatic treatment, which involves the use of antiemetics, antispasmodics, gastrointestinal protectants, and intravenous or subcutaneous fluids if dehydration is present.

2. Antibiotics to treat infectious diseases, throat infections, and food poisoning.

3. Treatment for shock (*see* Chapter 16, Emergency Care; Emergency Cases: Shock).

4. Treatment for poisonings (*see* Chapter 16, Emergency Care; Emergency Cases: Poisoning, Treatment).

5. Worming for parasites (*see* Chapter 2, Parasites; Internal Parasites: Treatment of Internal Parasites).

6. Treatment of liver and pancreatic diseases (*see* sections later in this chapter).

7. Treatment for kidney failure (*see* Chapter 11, The Urinary System; Kidney Disease: Treatment).

8. Surgical treatment for trauma, gastrointestinal tumors, intestinal obstruction, or foreign bodies.

9. Treatment of other diseases or disorders causing the vomiting.

Stomach Torsion and Dilation

Gastric (stomach) torsion, or twisting of the stomach, is preceded by bloating of the stomach from fluids, food, and gas. This is called gastric dilation, and frequently occurs in dogs, particularly in puppies that overeat. In itself, dilation is not usually serious, but if accompanied by gastric torsion, it is a life-threatening emergency. It occurs most frequently in large, deep-chested dogs and occasionally in small dogs. The exact cause of gastric torsion is unknown; many factors appear to be involved. A history of the dog having eaten a large quantity of food, particularly dry food, and drunk a lot of water before exercising precedes most cases.

SYMPTOMS In gastric dilation, the stomach swells, is painful, and the dog is restless and salivates excessively. In itself, this condition is not serious and is usually relieved by vomiting or the passage of gas. If, however, the gas-filled stomach becomes twisted, it will bloat even more, and the dog will try to vomit but will bring up nothing. Pain and restlessness will be evident, and will quickly lead to shock and death within twenty-four hours.

DIAGNOSIS   The diagnosis is made from the clinical signs, history of rapid onset, and evidence of a swollen, gas-filled stomach. X-rays are used to confirm the diagnosis.

TREATMENT   If the stomach is just dilated with gas but not twisted, inducing vomiting or introducing a stomach tube will give immediate relief.

If the dilation cannot be relieved by a stomach tube then immediate surgery gives the best chance for survival. The stomach is surgically untwisted and then sewn in the correct position to help prevent recurrences. Treatment for shock will also be essential. The success rate for this procedure is directly proportional to the speed with which the dog is treated.

Caution: If signs of stomach bloat occur, immediate veterinary treatment is essential; do not wait until morning if the symptoms occur at night. If you cannot get veterinary care, try giving the dog a large dose of an antacid such as Mylanta, and keep the dog walking. If this does not help, a dog owner can try to introduce a stomach tube (a garden hose can be used). If the hose will not go into the stomach, do not force it or you may perforate the esophagus. If all this fails, a last resort to save the dog's life is to use a sharp pointed instrument, such as a scissors, to puncture the stomach through the abdominal wall and release the gas. Veterinary care will be essential following this last procedure to prevent peritonitis.

PREVENTION   Dogs prone to stomach bloat or torsion should be fed small quantities of food and should not be allowed to drink excessively following eating. Dogs fed on dry food should have the food slightly moistened. No vigorous exercise should be allowed after feeding, nor should the dog be fed following exercises until he has had a rest.

Coprophagy (Stool Eating)

Stool eating is known technically as coprophagy. A more general term used to describe this is pica, which is defined as a perverted or depraved appetite for substances not ordinarily considered food. Stool eating is relatively common in young dogs, but its cause is not really known. There are many theoretical explanations, including boredom, a lack of digestive enzymes, an unbalanced diet, and vitamin and mineral deficiencies, especially the B vitamins. Dogs with gastritis (stomach upset), pancreatic disease, gum infections, or rabies often eat feces. So do teething puppies or those with stomach or intestinal parasites.

CONTROL Although feces contain some digestive enzymes, they also contain harmful bacteria and, very often, parasites. It is important, therefore, to try to control coprophagy in a dog. The following approaches are reported to have been successful in individual cases:

1. Disciplining the dog when it is seen eating stool. This is often all that is required. Care must be taken if disciplining is used for defecating in the house, as the dog may start to eat his stool to hide the evidence and thereby avoid punishment.

2. A change of diet to a different balanced dog food and more frequent feedings, plus the use of a vitamin-mineral supplement. This may control the problem if discipline does not help.

3. Adding the enzyme papain, which is present in meat tenderizer, to the dog's food (sprinkle it like salt on the food daily for one week). This may prevent coprophagy.

4. Adding glutamic acid to the dog's food. This is said to make the stools taste unpleasant to the dog. Glutamic acid capsules are available at drugstores; one after each meal or added to the food should be sufficient.

5. Adding carrots, pineapple, or pumpkin to the dog's food. They are also believed to make the stools distasteful to a dog.

6. Cleaning up the bowel movements at once. This is, of course, the most effective prevention.

7. Worming. This will take care of the problem if parasitic infestation is the cause.

COPROPHAGY MAY BE NORMAL BEHAVIOR FOR A DOG! An English veterinarian has recently completed studies on coprophagy in dogs, and his explanation and treatment appear valid. He believes that this behavior is a natural habit in canines, similar to that of rabbits, who consume their own feces in order to achieve more efficient absorption of nutrients from their diet. Unfortunately, most dog owners are aghast at this explanation and have difficulty in accepting such behavior as natural. In response to this reaction, the veterinarian developed a treatment technique which calls for the administration of a nausea-provoking drug (under veterinary supervision) to dogs shortly after they ingest feces. The dog then feels ill within ten minutes of eating the feces and makes a learned, unpleasant association with the item most recently consumed (the feces). The dog recovers in a few hours with no adverse effects and only an occasional dog needs more than one treatment. This same veterinarian concludes his research by making a plea to dog owners to accept this behavior when it occurs, to allow some of the vestigial wolf spirit—the hunter-scavenger—to remain alive!

Ulcers

An ulcer is an erosion or breaking down of the surface of an organ or tissue. Ulcers are not as common in dogs as they are in people, but they do occur on occasion in the lower esophagus, stomach, and duodenum (first part of the small intestine).

An increase in stomach acid and pepsin secretion can result in an ulcer in susceptible dogs, although not all ulcers are caused by high acid levels. In dogs, ulcers are more commonly associated with other conditions, such as kidney failure, liver disease, poisoning, corticosteroid drugs, and stomach cancer.

SYMPTOMS Many dogs with ulcers vomit a few hours after eating. There may also be signs of abdominal pain, weight loss, and anemia. Black, tarry stools are seen if the ulcer is bleeding. If an ulcer perforates into the abdominal cavity, immediate worsening of the symptoms, with evidence of severe pain, then collapse, will occur. This is an emergency situation and without treatment can be fatal in a few hours.

DIAGNOSIS The diagnosis of an ulcer is made by the history, clinical signs, and laboratory tests. It is confirmed by x-rays, and in some cases by using a gastroscope to visualize the ulcer and its location.

TREATMENT Because canine ulcers so frequently occur secondarily to other diseases, it is essential to treat the primary disease. Antacids, a bland diet, frequent feeding, and the use of some of the newer drugs for ulcer treatment, such as the histamine antagonist drug cimetidine, are all useful in treatment. Occasionally surgical intervention will be necessary.

INTESTINAL DISEASES AND DISORDERS

Diarrhea

Diarrhea is the passage of abnormally soft and frequent stools; it is not an uncommon problem in dogs. It results from inflammation of the small and/or large intestine, and these conditions are respectively called enteritis or colitis. If both intestines are involved the condition is called enterocolitis.

Common causes are: eating decomposed foods, or irritant (spicy) foods; overeating; a change in diet; eating a very rich diet containing a lot of meat or sugar; and food allergies. Occasionally, worms and nervousness may also cause diarrhea in dogs. More serious causes are severe food poisoning; bacterial and fungal intestinal infections; poisons; intestinal obstruction; tumors of the gastrointestinal tract; pancreatic disease; liver disease; kidney disease; infectious diseases such as distemper, canine infectious hepatitis, and leptospirosis; defective intestinal absorption; disease and disorders of the nervous system; shock; and trauma.

SYMPTOMS Most dogs have soft stool or diarrhea occasionally, but unless it recurs frequently or becomes chronic, treatment is unnecessary if the dog appears otherwise healthy.

If the diarrhea is accompanied by loss of appetite, depression, and dehydration, treatment is recommended. Foul-smelling, foamy diarrhea can be due to a lack of digestive enzymes from a diseased pancreas. Blood-tinged diarrhea or black, tarry stools indicate bleeding in the upper gastrointestinal tract; these are signs of serious gastrointestinal disease and require treatment. Light colored, soft stools may indicate liver disease.

DIAGNOSIS Diagnosis is made by the history, a physical examination, laboratory examination of the stool, and other laboratory tests. X-rays can be helpful diagnostically in some cases.

TREATMENT *Home treatment.* To treat diarrhea in a dog at home, do not allow it to eat or drink for twenty-four hours. Give Kaopectate at a dosage of 1 teaspoon per 10 pounds of body weight every six hours, unless this makes the dog vomit. After twenty-four hours feed a small portion of a bland diet such as baby food, rice, a boiled egg, or a little lean cooked beef or chicken, or use a homemade diet (*see* Chapter 1, Nutrition; Types of Diets for Dogs: Gastrointestinal Upset Diet). At this time allow the dog a limited amount of water. Continue to feed the bland diet with water every six hours for two to three days, then gradually get the dog back on its normal diet while allowing it free access to water again. A special canned food formulated for dogs with diarrhea, called Prescription Diet i/d made by Hill's, is available from veterinarians.

If the dog owner suspects the diarrhea is related to specific foods, then the problem could be a food allergy. Eliminate these foods from the diet or change the diet completely but gradually, and see if this alleviates the diarrhea problem (*see* Chapter 3, Allergies; Food Allergies).

Veterinary treatment. If these home treatments do not clear up the problem, or if the dog is seriously ill or in poor condition, it is best to see a veterinarian. The veterinarian will probably be able to determine the cause of the diarrhea, although this is not always possible if the condition is of a chronic nature. Even in chronic cases, treatment can be helpful. Be sure to bring a sample of the dog's stool to the veterinary hospital and to tell the veterinarian as much as possible about the nature of the problem.

Veterinary treatments will vary depending on the cause and severity of the diarrhea, but are generally similar to the treatments outlined for vomiting.

Flatulence

Flatulence is the presence of excessive quantities of air or gases in the stomach or intestines. A flatulent dog in the house can be quite embarrassing!

Flatulence is due to excessive gas formation from the bacterial breakdown of food or from swallowing too much air, usually while eating.

Gas-producing foods, such as beans, root vegetables, cabbage, cauliflower, and onions, should be avoided. Milk causes digestive problems in some dogs. Rich, high-protein meat diets may also cause this problem. Diets containing rich carbohydrates have also been incriminated in people, but are less likely to be the cause in dogs. Foods that cause flatulence in one dog may not in another.

TREATMENT Avoiding gas-producing foods should help. A change of diet should assist a dog owner in identifying what is giving the dog flatulence. Cat foods should not be fed to dogs prone to flatulence, since cat foods are higher in meat protein than dog foods. Few dogs have problems with gas when fed exclusively on dry dog foods.

Constipation

Constipation is difficult or infrequent passage of stools. The causes include eating excessive quantities of bones; eating dry food and not drinking enough water; tumors of the gastrointestinal tract or other abdominal tumors pressing on the intestines; an enlarged prostate gland; large numbers of intestinal parasites blocking the intestines; foreign bodies in the intestinal tract, causing obstruction; trauma; diseases and disorders of the nervous system; not enough exercise; old age; and obesity.

SYMPTOMS   The symptoms are infrequent, hard stools and straining to defecate. More serious signs are loss of appetite, vomiting, and depression. It is important for a dog owner not to confuse constipation with straining related to urinary tract diseases.

DIAGNOSIS   The history is diagnostic and a veterinarian can usually palpate the hard stools in the bowel.

TREATMENT   If constipation is due to another disease or disorder, the primary problem will also need to be treated. Treatment of constipation involves the use of enemas, stool softeners, and laxatives. If the constipation cannot be resolved by these treatments, it may be necessary to anesthetize the dog and crush and remove the stool with forceps.

PREVENTION   Foods that cause constipation should be avoided. Dogs prone to this problem should be encouraged to drink more and be exercised more vigorously and frequently. An obese dog should be put on a reducing diet. Stool softeners may be recommended by the veterinarian on a long-term basis for chronic cases. Mild laxatives such as mineral oil can be used when needed, but should not be given on a continuing basis. Stool-bulking agents and additional fiber in the diet may help in some cases.

ANAL SAC DISEASE

The anal sacs are pouches located on each side of the anus. These sacs are lined with glandular cells which secrete a brownish oily fluid, which is discharged through a single duct

from each sac during defecation. These anal sacs were probably used as a spraying defense mechanism by the ancestors of
today's dog, similar to the skunk's spray. Dogs often empty
these anal sacs when frightened.

The anal sacs may become impacted and/or infected. If the
ducts become blocked, the sacs become swollen with secretions which then become hardened or impacted, and this
often develops into an abscess. Streptococcal or staphylococcal organisms can infect the anal sacs, causing an anal saccu-
litis (inflammation). Why some dogs have these problems is
not known, but the problem is associated with abnormal
bowel function, thick gland secretions, small ducts, and poor
muscle tone as is found in obese dogs. Anal sac problems are
common in Chihuahuas and poodles.

SYMPTOMS If the ducts become blocked or the sacs become overfilled or infected, the secretion develops a disagree-
able odor. Because of the pain and irritation that result, the
dog may scoot his bottom along the floor, and lick and bite
constantly at the area around the anus. A moist dermatitis
(skin condition) may result from this self-inflicted trauma.
Pain will be most noticeable during defecation.

DIAGNOSIS Diagnosis is made by the history and symptoms.

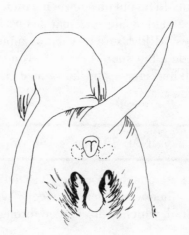

Anal Sacs

TREATMENT   The veterinarian can gently express and empty impacted anal sacs by placing a gloved index finger into the rectum and a thumb on the other side of the sac and then compressing the sac between these fingers. Since the problem of impacted anal sacs tends to recur, the veterinarian can show a dog owner how to perform this procedure by pressing on either side of the sacs while covering the duct with cotton to collect the secretion. Depending on the severity of the problem, this may need to be done on a weekly or monthly schedule.

If the anal sacs are infected, surgical drainage, followed by instillation of antibiotics into these cavities, may be necessary. Severely infected cases, or chronically recurring impacted cases, may call for surgical removal of the sacs.

LIVER DISEASE

The liver is the largest organ of the body, performing more essential body functions than any other organ. It also has remarkable regenerative capacity and can continue to perform without signs of disease when only about 25% of it is functioning. The liver produces bile, which is stored in the gallbladder and aids in the digestion of fat. It is also involved in carbohydrate, fat, and protein metabolism; in detoxification, inactivation, and excretion of many natural and poisonous products; in manufacturing some enzymes, vitamins, and other essential nutrients; and in producing a number of blood coagulation factors.

Inflammation of the liver is called hepatitis. The primary causes of liver disease in dogs are poisons; infectious viral, bacterial, and fungal diseases; parasites; tumors; nutritional deficiencies; allergic and immune system disorders; and trauma.

SYMPTOMS   The symptoms of liver disease are often nonspecific, and depend on the cause, severity of damage to the organ, the presence of other disease, and the length of the illness. The symptoms include some or all of the following:

- Swelling of the abdomen and abdominal discomfort, which may or may not be painful. The swelling is due to increase in size of the liver and fluid accumulation in the abdominal cavity.
- Digestive disorders, such as nausea, vomiting, loss of appetite, indigestion, and flatulence.
- Weight loss.
- Weakness, usually accompanied by depression. Occasionally, hyperactivity can occur if the cause is due to poisoning or nervous system disorders.
- Fever, particularly if the cause is an infectious agent.
- Anemia and bleeding tendencies.
- Poor haircoat and skin condition.
- Jaundice, which causes yellowing of the skin and body tissues from bile pigment deposits.
- Change in color of feces which may be light colored or darker than normal.
- Change in color of the urine which may be darker, foamy, and have a greenish tinge.

DIAGNOSIS The diagnosis of liver disease is made by the history, clinical signs, a physical examination, and blood and urine tests. There are a number of liver function tests that may be required to determine the type and degree of damage. X-rays and biopsies are sometimes required to confirm the diagnosis or determine the cause.

TREATMENT Elimination of the cause, if this is possible, is the first aim of treatment in liver disease. There is no medical cure for liver disease, so treatment is directed at supportive care and treating the symptoms, both of which allow the liver to heal itself. Rest is essential, and a dog may have to be confined to ensure this. Serious cases will require intravenous fluids and feeding. Antibiotics are used in most cases, particularly in those due to infectious diseases. Special diets that lessen the load on the liver will be recommended if the dog is eating. Extra vitamins, particularly the B vitamins, and digestive aid drugs may be used. Most drugs must be used with caution in liver disease, as the liver is no longer able to break them down and as a result, they may be toxic to the liver and lead to even further liver damage. The aim of treatment is to keep the dog alive during the critical stage of liver disease, so that the liver can repair and regenerate; if the liver can achieve this, most dogs will recover without serious impairment.

PANCREATIC DISEASE

The two main functions of the pancreas are the production of insulin, which is passed into the blood to aid in the utilization of sugars, and the production of enzymes that are passed into the duodenum (the first part of the small intestine) for the digestion of fats, carbohydrates, and proteins.

Inflammation of the pancreas is called pancreatitis, but the exact cause in dogs is unknown. It is associated with obesity, poor nutrition, trauma, and tumors. Obstruction of the bile or pancreatic ducts can also lead to pancreatitis. Bacterial infections are not a primary cause, but can complicate pancreatitis once it has occurred.

SYMPTOMS   Pancreatitis can be acute or chronic. The signs of acute disease are:

- Sudden onset.
- Severe abdominal pain—the dog will be reluctant to move and will stand with an arched back, and tensed abdomen.
- Vomiting that occurs some hours after eating (rather than immediately, which is more diagnostic of acute gastritis).
- Diarrhea.
- Dehydration.

- Depression.
- Collapse and shock.

The signs of chronic or less severe disease are:

- Increased thirst.
- Excessive urination.
- Bulky, fatty, foul-smelling grey stools, particularly after a high-fat meal is fed.
- Loss of weight.
- Occasional nausea, vomiting, flatulence, and other signs of digestive upsets.
- Poor general condition, particularly of the skin and hair-coat.
- Signs of diabetes mellitus in progressive cases (*see* Chapter 14, Infectious, Respiratory, and Hormonal Diseases; Endocrine (Hormonal) System Diseases and Disorders: Diabetes Mellitus).

DIAGNOSIS Diagnosis is made from the history, the clinical signs, a physical examination, and confirmed by laboratory tests on the blood, urine, and feces. X-rays can be helpful in diagnosis.

TREATMENT Acute pancreatitis needs emergency treatment for shock. Antibiotics and pain-relief drugs will also be necessary. No food can be given by mouth, so intravenous fluids and feeding will be part of the treatment. Some cases will require surgical intervention if this will reverse the cause.

PROGNOSIS The prognosis is generally not good for acute pancreatitis, although up to 50% of affected dogs can be saved with early treatment. Some cases tend to recur and become chronic, and require careful watching for symptoms and feeding of a special diet available from veterinarians. Pancreatic extracts and vitamins will also be part of the chronic case's treatment and are often needed for the rest of the dog's life.

In either the acute or chronic disease, if the pancreas is severely damaged, the dog will become diabetic.

11

The Urinary System

KIDNEY FUNCTION AND FAILURE

Diseases affecting the kidneys are among the most common medical problems seen in dogs, particularly old dogs.

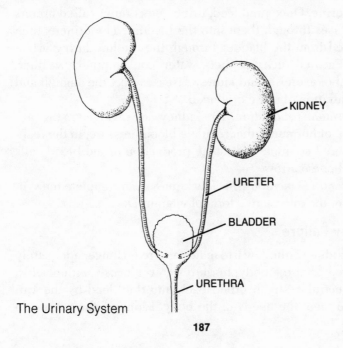

KIDNEY

URETER

BLADDER

URETHRA

The Urinary System

(Males are affected more than females.) To understand kidney disease it is necessary to know the function of the kidneys and what occurs when they fail.

Kidney Function

The main functions of the kidney are:

Excretion. The blood in the body passes through the kidneys, and waste materials, water, and other body chemicals are removed from the blood by the kidneys. The waste materials and excess water are then excreted as urine.

Regulation. The kidneys also regulate the levels of many constituents of the blood, reabsorbing back into the blood the water, sugars, amino acids, and electrolytes (such as sodium, potassium, and chloride) needed by the body.

Urine production. Depending on the body's needs, the kidneys return to the blood up to 99% of the water and useful chemical constituents. The remaining percentage, composed of waste materials, excess water, and excess electrolytes, forms urine. Once produced, urine enters tubes called ureters and passes through them into the bladder. The urine is then expelled from the bladder through the urethra during urination. Factors such as diet, water consumption, weather, amount of exercise, and kidney disease affect the amount and concentration of urine produced.

Hormone production. The kidneys are involved in the production of hormones that regulate blood pressure, in the reabsorption of sodium, and in the production of red blood cells in the bone marrow.

Vitamin D metabolism. The kidneys can complete the synthesis of the most active form of vitamin D.

Kidney Failure

In kidney failure, waste materials are no longer adequately removed from the body, nor are water, glucose, amino acids, and electrolytes reabsorbed back into the blood by the kidneys to meet the needs of the body. Kidney failure signs do not occur until about three-quarters of the kidney tissue is damaged. Kidney failure can be either compensated or uncompensated.

Compensated kidney failure. In early kidney failure the dog can compensate or adjust to the failure by drinking more water, which leads to a larger volume of more dilute urine. While this allows the waste materials to be flushed out of the body, some of the needed chemical constituents are also lost. The signs of compensated kidney failure are increased thirst, increased urination (in both frequency and quantity), weight loss, digestive upsets that may include periodic vomiting or diarrhea, and a dry, flaky skin.

Uncompensated kidney failure. When kidney failure is severe, either due to an acute kidney disease or to worsening of a chronic condition, and the dog can no longer compensate by drinking and urinating excessively, the kidney failure is called uncompensated. This results in a serious condition called uremia, in which poisonous wastes accumulate in the body and the electrolytes in the body become unbalanced. Uremia is a serious medical condition and without prompt treatment can prove fatal. Early signs are increased thirst, vomiting, low temperature, listlessness, and little or no urine. Later signs are depression, excess urine, dehydration, pain, weakness, muscle twitching, coma, and convulsions, leading to death. If the onset of uremia is slow, signs will include loss of appetite, weight loss, reddened eyes, bad breath, mouth ulcers, discolored tongue, anemia, bone thinning, and skin disorders.

KIDNEY DISEASE

There are numerous causes of kidney disease, but all of them can lead to severe kidney damage, and then to kidney failure. The failure may be acute (sudden), or it may take years to develop, a condition referred to as chronic kidney failure.

If an animal suffers acute kidney failure and survives, the condition may become chronic if the kidney damage cannot be reversed. Inflammation of the kidneys is called nephritis, and there are other complicated technical names for various forms of kidney diseases, but, in general terms, the causes of most kidney failures in dogs are congenital or hereditary defects; bacterial and viral infections; injury; abscesses; poisons; parasites; kidney stones; immune system abnormalities; tumors; and shock.

SYMPTOMS   (*See* Kidney Failure, above.)

DIAGNOSIS   While it is not always possible to determine the cause of kidney disease, particularly if the disease is chronic, the following approach to diagnosis allows the veterinarian to determine if the dog's kidneys are failing, the degree of damage to the kidneys, the best method of treatment, and the prognosis.

1. *Medical history.* A detailed description of the dog's medical history, with emphasis on the recent appetite, water consumption, urine output, and appearance of the urine will aid the veterinarian in making a diagnosis of kidney disease.

2. *Physical examination.* The veterinarian will conduct a complete physical examination of the dog and palpate the abdomen to discover any obvious abnormalities of the kidneys or bladder.

3. *Urinalysis.* A urine sample will be collected either during urination, by manual expression of the bladder, or by passing a catheter. Numerous tests can be conducted on the urine to aid in diagnosing kidney disease and in determining the extent of the disease. If infection is present, bacteria can be seen on microscopic examination of the urine, and a culture and sensitivity test of a urine sample should be conducted to determine which antibiotic to use in treatment.

4. *Blood tests.* Blood tests can aid in diagnosing infections, anemia, the extent to which the kidneys are disposing of the

body's waste materials, and the balance of the electrolytes in the body.

5. *Kidney function tests.* There are a number of tests to measure the degree of kidney function, and some of these tests may be advisable if there is serious kidney failure evident.

6. *X-rays.* X-rays can be helpful in diagnosing some kidney diseases, or to observe the kidneys during some of the kidney function tests.

7. *Biopsy.* Removal of tissues for microscopic examination is done in kidney disease to confirm a diagnosis or to eliminate a suspected diagnosis. It is particularly useful in diagnosing tumors. A biopsy can be done with a special biopsy punch needle inserted through the skin using a local anesthetic and sedation, or during exploratory surgery under full anesthesia.

TREATMENT Acute kidney failure requires immediate hospital care. Chronic kidney failure requires routine veterinary examinations, but most of the treatment and care is done by the dog owner at home. Since chronic kidney failure can progress slowly to acute failure as the disease worsens, the dog owner must be alert to signs of acute failure.

Acute kidney failure treatment. Treatment for acute kidney failure requires some or all of the following approaches:

1. Intravenous or subcutaneous fluids to restore the water and electrolyte balance.

2. Antibiotics to treat infections.

3. An antidote if available, if poisoning is involved.

4. Sedatives and pain killers if required. Tranquilizers are frequently used to prevent vomiting.

5. Cortisone and other drugs if the dog is in shock.

6. Blood transfusions.

7. Provided that the dog is not vomiting, a special low-protein, high-calorie diet is given; if the dog is not eating, such a diet should be administered by stomach tube.

8. Vitamin B injections.

9. Surgery in cases where such intervention can be curative; performed rarely if kidney failure is evident, as both kidneys are then always involved.

The use of an artificial kidney machine, peritoneal lavage, and kidney transplants are not routine in veterinary medicine, but can be done by some veterinary hospitals. Less expensive portable artificial kidney machines are now being developed and many veterinary hospitals have or will have this equipment. Like artificial kidney machines, peritoneal lavage removes waste materials from the body. It is done by injecting large volumes of a special fluid into the dog's abdominal cavity and removing it in a few hours, after it has absorbed the waste materials the failing kidneys cannot handle. Kidney transplants have been done on dogs, but the problems of finding matched tissues and rejection are the same as those in human medicine.

These three techniques involve extensive care and considerable expense, but are available to dog owners if they want them. If a veterinary hospital cannot supply these procedures, ask for a referral or contact the university veterinary department of the closest veterinary school.

While acute kidney failure is a critical situation, many dogs can be saved with intensive veterinary care. Some will fully recover kidney function and will need no further treatment; others will be left with chronic kidney failure and will need continuing care.

Chronic kidney failure treatment. Although there is no cure for chronic kidney failure, treatment can prolong a dog's life for many years. The dog can be kept relatively healthy and happy, without too much inconvenience or expense for the owner. The objectives of treatment are to help the failing kidneys eliminate waste materials by controlling and monitoring liquid intake, to decrease the amount of waste material the kidneys need to eliminate by using diet control, and to replace the chemical constituents needed by the body which are lost in the increased amount of urine. In other words, the aim of treatment is to keep the dog with chronic kidney failure in a compensated condition and to prevent uremia developing. This is done by the following means:

1. The dog is encouraged to drink lots of fluids to maintain a high urine output, which helps to flush out waste materials from the body. The dog should not be made to retain its urine for long periods of time.

2. The sodium lost in the urine is replaced with table salt, salt tablets, or sodium bicarbonate. If the dog has heart disease, however, salt should not be used without close veterinary supervision. Current research information indicates that, in fact, salt should *not* be used to treat most dogs suffering from kidney failure.

3. Since protein produces most of the waste material that the kidneys excrete, and dogs must have some protein to live, it is essential to feed the smallest amount of the highest quality protein to maintain the dog in good condition. A number of special diets, such as Prescription Diets k/d and u/d made by Hill's, which have been designed specifically for dogs with kidney disease, are available from the veterinarian. These diets reduce the demands on the kidneys by producing a minimum of protein waste. Dogs with kidney disease must remain on these diets for life, although some adjustments may need to be made in the protein intake as the kidney disease advances. Another alternative is to feed a homemade diet (*see* Chapter 1, Nutrition; Types of Diets for Dogs: Kidney Failure Diet).

4. Water soluble vitamins lost in the urine need to be replaced. Supplements high in the B complex vitamins and vitamin C will be required.

5. Anabolic steroids, drugs which stimulate the appetite and reduce the demands on the kidneys, may be given.

Stress or any sudden change in routine must be avoided. Other medical problems should be treated promptly, and the teeth, in particular, should be attended to. Routine hospital visits and tests will be required to check the dog's progress and make adjustments in treatments if required. Any signs of deterioration, uremia, or acute kidney failure episodes should be treated at once.

Kidney failure is progressive, but in dogs, and especially old dogs, it tends to progress slowly in most cases; with care these dogs can live for many years. Eventually, even with the most careful treatment, the dog will no longer be able to compensate for the failing kidneys, and uremia will develop. The veterinarian, with the aid of laboratory tests, can usually tell when the condition has become irreversible, even with further extensive treatments, and it is at this point that euthanasia should be considered. It is a good idea to discuss this with the veterinarian ahead of time, as it is much more difficult to make this decision in a time of crisis. For the dog with failing kidneys, there is a point when life is no longer worth living, and a slow, painful death is ahead, so a decision for euthanasia needs to be made to avoid prolonged suffering by the dog.

BLADDER AND URINARY TRACT DISEASES

Cystitis (Bladder Inflammation)

Cystitis is an acute or chronic inflammation of the bladder that damages the bladder wall and causes mucus, blood, and other organic debris to accumulate in the bladder. The cause of cystitis is, in most cases, a bacterial infection, which reaches the bladder generally from the lower urinary or genital tract, but can also descend from a kidney infection into the bladder, or from an infection elsewhere in the body via the blood.

There are a number of factors which predispose a dog to cystitis, and these include:

- Urine retention due to narrowing of the urethra from calculi (stones), trauma, or tumors. Bacteria grow more readily in urine which is retained or stagnant.
- Urine retention due to damage to the nerve supply to the bladder from spinal cord lesions such as slipped discs, infections, or tumors.
- Urine retention due to congenital defects of the bladder.
- Urine retention from dogs forced to hold urine for long periods.
- Deficiencies of fluids and vitamin A.
- Diabetes mellitus or other causes of sugar in the urine, resulting in a good medium for bacterial growth.
- Trauma to the bladder from accidents.

SYMPTOMS The symptoms of cystitis are increased frequency of urination, sometimes with evidence of straining or pain. The urine may be bloody, particularly the urine expelled at the end of urination. While actual blood is not always seen, in most cases of cystitis there is blood in the urine, which gives the urine a pinkish tinge. Otherwise, the dog is usually alert, with normal appetite and temperature. If the dog cannot urinate at all due to obstruction of the urethra or nerve damage to the bladder, then signs of uremia will be evident, and immediate treatment is essential. Cystitis is more frequent in female dogs, but more serious in males. This is because the female urethra is wide and seldom becomes blocked with stones, whereas in the male the urethra cannot dilate as much and readily becomes blocked.

DIAGNOSIS The history and clinical signs lead to a diagnosis of cystitis. Urinalysis will confirm the diagnosis, and if bacteria are evident, culture and sensitivity testing will be recommended in most cases to determine the antibiotic to use in treatment. If the primary cause of the cystitis cannot be determined, x-rays and even a biopsy may be required. Another technique helpful in diagnosing the cause of cystitis in difficult cases is cystoscopy, in which a special instrument is used to inspect the lower urinary tract.

TREATMENT The first approach to treating cystitis in dogs is to remove the predisposing causes, which may entail surgery if calculi, tumors, or trauma are involved; if diabetes mellitus is also present, it should be treated at the same time.

Most cystitis cases are caused by bacterial infections, and antibiotics are effective in clearing them up. Some cases will require long-term treatments; a number of different antibiotics may be tried before an effective one is found. Antispasmotics, pain relievers, and urinary antiseptics are used initially in severe cases to relieve the symptoms. Urinary acidifiers—such as ammonium chloride, methionine, mandelic acid, and vitamin C—are given, often for years if recurrences occur. (Most of the bacteria that cause cystitis in dogs do not grow well in acid urine.)

To prevent urinary stagnation, the dog owner should salt the dog's food, as this leads to increased drinking and increased urination, both of which help to keep the bladder flushed out. The dog with cystitis should never be allowed to hold urine, but should have free access to the outdoors and be encouraged to urinate frequently.

Most cases of cystitis can be cleared up with treatment. Recurrences are not uncommon, and some cases become chronic and require continuing treatment to prevent the infection spreading to the kidneys. Following a course of treatment, urinalysis should be done to be sure the infection is under control, and dog owners should watch closely for signs of recurrences, so early retreatment may be started.

Urolithiasis (Urinary Stones)

Urolithiasis is the formation of urinary calculi, also called uroliths or stones. These stones are found mostly in the bladder, but can also locate in the kidneys or the urethra. Why these stones form is unknown, although certain breeds of dogs are affected more often than others; this points to a hereditary predisposition. Stagnation of urine is also a predisposing factor. There are four types of uroliths or stones found in dogs. They are:

1. *Phosphate calculi.* About 75% of urinary stones found in dogs are of this type. They are white or grey, chalky, and form in alkaline urine. They are often referred to as triple phosphates because they are made up of magnesium, ammonium, and calcium, together with phosphate.

2. *Urate calculi.* These account for about 10% of all urinary stones found in dogs. They are small, hard, oval-shaped, and tan or yellow in color. They occur most often in the Dalmatian breed, which has an inherited characteristic of excreting large amounts of uric acid in the urine.

3. *Cystine calculi.* These comprise about 5% of urinary stones, and are found predominantly in dachshunds, Dalmatians, and some terrier breeds. The stones are small, smooth, round, and yellowish.

4. *Oxalate calculi.* These usually single, hard, prickly, egg-shaped, white stones account for about 10% of urinary stones in dogs.

SYMPTOMS   Most urinary calculi are located in the bladder, and the symptoms are the same as those for cystitis: frequent urination and blood in the urine. If the stones are located in the urethra, the signs are more acute and include urine dribbling or no urine, a tense distended abdomen, pain, straining to urinate; if prolonged, signs of uremia occur. Kidney stones do not show signs until kidney damage is severe unless they enter and block the ureter, and acute signs of uremia develop.

DIAGNOSIS   Diagnosis is made by the history and a physical examination by the veterinarian, who can often feel the stones in the bladder. Urinary stones are confirmed by urinalysis and x-rays.

TREATMENT   Most calculi have to be removed surgically. Phosphate calculi are often associated with cystitis, so treatment for this disease will also be required. Stones blocking the urethra can usually be pushed back into the bladder with a catheter and then removed surgically.

PREVENTION Up to 20% of urinary calculi recur, so preventive measures are essential in affected dogs. These vary, depending on the type of stones.

Phosphate calculi form in alkaline urine and are associated with cystitis, so urinary acidifiers, salt to increase drinking and urination, and treating and preventing recurrences of cystitis are all essential preventive measures. A special diet, Prescription Diet, s/d, made by Hill's, is now available from veterinarians; it not only helps prevent recurrence of phosphate calculi but has also been used successfully to dissolve calculi and thereby avoid surgical removal. This diet has a low protein and mineral content and an increased level of salt, and produces an acid urine.

Urate calculi preventive measures include additional salt in the diet, treating infection if present, and the use of sodium bicarbonate to keep the urine alkaline, as these calculi are more soluble in alkaline urine.

Cystine calculi preventive measures are the same as those for urate calculi, and additionally a low-protein diet is recommended. Some experimental drugs are being studied to prevent recurrences of these stones.

Oxalate calculi preventive measures include the use of salt and treating any cystitis present.

Urinary Incontinence

Urinary incontinence is an inability to control urination, either due to overflow of urine or loss of bladder control. There are many causes of urinary incontinence. One relatively common cause is from paralysis of the bladder due to spinal cord damage from slipped discs, infections, tumors, congenital defects, or accidents. In these cases the bladder overdistends and then dribbles urine because the nerves no longer stimulate the bladder to contract and empty. Other causes of incontinence are damage to the bladder itself from accidents, obstruction of the urethra, estrogen deficiency in older spayed female dogs, and as a secondary effect of cystitis in which there is urine stagnation.

TREATMENT   If the cause can be eliminated, the incontinence will clear up (*see* specific disease for treatment). However, if there is bladder paralysis from damage to the nervous system, the bladder will have to be expressed manually a few times a day, or catheterized. Dogs with bladder paralysis from nervous system damage should be given a few months to see if the condition can be reversed, as it may take that long before the nerve tissue repairs itself.

12

The Nervous System

The nervous system is the communication network of the body; it regulates and controls nearly all body functions, such as the senses, memory, muscle movements, heartbeat, respiration, and digestive secretions. It is made up of the central

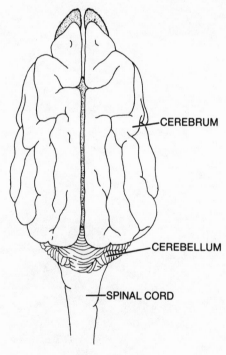

The Brain (Top View)

and the peripheral nervous systems. The central nervous system includes the brain within the skull and the spinal cord within the vertebral column. The peripheral nervous system includes the twelve cranial nerves, which exit from the brain, and, in the dog, thirty-six or thirty-seven pairs of spinal nerves, each of which has an outgoing, or motor, root and an incoming, or sensory, root. The twelve cranial nerves control the muscles of the face, hearing, smell, sight, taste, and also include a major nerve, called the vagus nerve, which goes to many organs of the chest and abdomen. The spinal nerves control all other areas of the body. The brain and spinal cord float in cerebrospinal fluid, which helps to protect and cushion them against injury.

DISEASES AND DISORDERS OF THE BRAIN

Epilepsy

An epileptic dog suffers from recurring brain seizures, more commonly known as fits or convulsions—regardless of cause. Although many diseases cause brain seizures, only *recurring* seizures are called epilepsy. Epilepsy is only a symptom of a malfunction of the brain, not a disease; it results from a transient electrical activity disturbance of brain function.

There are two types of epilepsy in dogs:

Idiopathic epilepsy (of unknown cause): Idiopathic epilepsy is a functional disorder of the brain in which no cause can be found. Some types of idiopathic epilepsy in dogs are inherited, but the genetic transmission is not fully understood. It occurs more commonly in certain breeds of dogs—cocker spaniels, German shepherds, Saint Bernards, Irish setters, poodles, and beagles.

Acquired epilepsy. Acquired epilepsy arises from a structural abnormality or organic disease of the brain. Some causes are congenital or birth injury; trauma; brain tumors; encephalitis (brain infection); cardiovascular disease; poisonings; parasites; canine distemper; lack of oxygen; liver disease; hydrocephalus; low blood sugar; and low blood calcium.

SYMPTOMS Epileptic seizures have three phases. The first phase, referred to as the "aura," occurs prior to the seizure. The dog appears dazed and will exhibit such signs as restlessness, nervousness, shaking, whining, salivation, aimless wandering, hiding, and personality changes. This phase can last from a few seconds to a few days and often goes unnoticed by the owner.

The second phase is the actual seizure; it can be focal or generalized. If focal, only one part of the body is affected; an ear, lip, or leg may shake. If generalized, there is a staring appearance to the eyes, and the dog stiffens, falls on its side, and the legs make running motions. The dog may yelp, froth at the mouth, and empty its bowels and bladder; it may also lose consciousness. Usually only a few of these symptoms occur. This second phase may last anywhere from a few seconds to five minutes. If the seizure lasts longer than that, it is called "status epilepticus," which means continuous seizures; this can be fatal without emergency medical treatment.

The third phase is recovery. The dog may appear confused, disoriented, and sleepy. Pacing, walking in circles, hiding, and other changes in personality are not unusual in this phase, which can last from a few minutes to a few days.

Although frightening for a dog owner to watch, seizures are not thought to be painful for the dog, since the movements and sounds are made involuntarily. A dog should not be moved or handled during a seizure except to prevent it from injuring itself. Dogs do not tend to swallow their tongues, so the dog owner should not put his or her fingers in the dog's mouth during a seizure lest a bad bite result. Talking to the dog and stroking it may help.

Epileptic seizures due to heredity usually start between one and five years of age in dogs. Initially, the seizures tend to be mild; they increase in severity over several years and may then become stable or decrease in severity. There is a great deal of variability in the course of epilepsy in dogs. Acquired epilepsy can start at any age.

DIAGNOSIS   The medical history of the dog and a detailed description of the type and frequency of the seizures will aid the veterinarian in making a diagnosis of epilepsy. A thorough physical and neurological examination, blood tests, and in some cases a cerebrospinal fluid tap, electroencephalogram (a tracing of the electrical activity of the brain), or brain x-rays may be required to determine if the seizures are being caused by structural or organic brain disease. If no specific cause can be found, idiopathic epilepsy is diagnosed.

TREATMENT   If a cause for epileptic seizures can be found, then treatment is directed at removing the cause.

Epilepsy is treated with anticonvulsant drugs. Four drugs, either alone or in combination, are commonly used: diphenyl-hydantoin (Dilantin), primidone, phenobarbital, and diazepam (Valium). The dosage is related to the frequency and severity of the seizures. It may take months, using a number of drugs or drug combinations, to control seizures in some cases. Even well-controlled epileptic dogs will have one or two seizures a year. If no convulsions occur for a year, the veterinarian may slowly reduce the drug dosage. Some dogs can be gradually taken off the medication completely, but most dogs must remain on it for life. About 30% of dogs do not respond to treatment.

Owners of epileptic dogs should be told that their dogs must not be given antihistamines and tranquilizers of the phenothiazine group of drugs because these drugs may bring on a seizure.

Dogs with epilepsy should lead a regular life, and should not be exposed to stress which may bring on a seizure. Because it is sometimes difficult to determine if epilepsy is acquired or inherited, dogs with epilepsy should not be used for breeding and should, preferably, be neutered.

204 The Nervous System

Hydrocephalus

Hydrocephalus directly translated means water (hydro) and head (cephalus). It is a condition in which an abnormal amount of fluid accumulates within the cranial vault of the skull. In a young dog it is accompanied by enlargement of the head, which becomes dome shaped, and an opening on the top of the skull, called a soft spot.

The fluid accumulation in hydrocephalus arises from an excessive amount of cerebrospinal fluid, due to overproduction of the fluid, obstruction of fluid flow, inadequate reabsorption of fluid, or a combination of these. The condition can be congenital (present at birth); these cases are usually due to a hereditary defect, seen most often in small breeds, such as the Chihuahua, Pekingese, and Boston terrier.

Hydrocephalus can also be acquired secondarily to other brain injuries, most commonly brain infections, traumas, brain tumors, and poisonings.

SYMPTOMS Many cases of hydrocephalus show no obvious signs. Others show only the dome-shaped head and the soft spot. Still others progress to a point where some or all of the following signs may occur:

- Irritability.
- Depression.
- Awkward gait.
- Knuckling of the feet.
- Paralysis.
- Loss of vision.
- Excessive sleeping.
- Seizures.

DIAGNOSIS Diagnosis is made by the history, clinical signs, and a physical examination; it can be confirmed by x-rays in most cases.

TREATMENT Medical treatment involves the use of diuretic drugs (to remove the excess fluid), together with corticosteroids (to reduce the swelling and inflammation). Surgical treatment involves draining off the excess fluid by inserting temporary or permanent drain tubes. The prognosis, even with treatment, is not good, and most cases are progressive once serious neurological symptoms occur.

PREVENTION   A dome-shaped skull is one of the major signs of hydrocephalus, and many breeders deliberately breed for this characteristic. Also, the soft spot, or hole, in the top of the skull is seen in many of these same dogs, and this, too, is abnormal, although accepted by breeders of dogs such as Chihuahuas and Pekingese as a normal characteristic. As a result, hydrocephalus is on the increase in certain breeds of dogs today. Many of these dogs will never show clinical signs of hydrocephalus and can live out a normal life span. Unfortunately, this leads breeders to believe that the dome-shaped skull and soft spot are not abnormal or a serious hazard. The defect is being propagated by breeding, and such dogs are at risk of developing progressive signs of hydrocephalus during their lifetime. Such breeding practices should be stopped to prevent hereditary hydrocephalus.

Senility

Senility is defined as the physical and mental deterioration associated with old age. Senility does occur in dogs, but compared to its occurrence in people, it is rare. One of the most common causes of senility in people is arteriosclerosis which leads to narrowing of the blood vessels of the brain. The blood supply to the brain is then inadequate for normal function. This condition is relatively rare in dogs.

There are other less common, age-related causes of brain degeneration in people and dogs that can lead to senility.

SYMPTOMS   Signs of senility in dogs include reduced response to stimuli, irritability, forgetfulness, confusion, and sleepiness.

DIAGNOSIS   If an older, otherwise healthy dog has these symptoms, and the severity of the symptoms does not increase rapidly (which would indicate other neurological causes, such as a brain tumor), senility is most likely the cause. Other neurological tests, laboratory tests, and x-rays may be necessary to rule out other brain diseases.

TREATMENT   Senility in dogs is a slow process. At present there is no effective treatment, although various drugs and geriatric products may help mask the symptoms.

Encephalitis

Encephalitis is an inflammation or infection of the brain. The causes of encephalitis are viral, bacterial, and fungal infections, and trauma. In the dog, the most common causes are canine distemper or the rabies virus. Bacterial and fungal infections often spread from infection sites in other areas of the body via the bloodstream, or from a sinus or internal ear infection.

SYMPTOMS   The symptoms of encephalitis are quite variable, and depending on the severity of the inflammation, include some or all of the following:

- Fever.
- Head pain.
- Vomiting.
- Diarrhea.
- Weakness.
- Depression.
- Blindness.
- Paralysis.
- Convulsions (seizures).
- Coma.

DIAGNOSIS   Diagnosis is made by the symptoms, a physical and neurological examination, and laboratory blood tests; sometimes x-rays and an examination of the cerebrospinal fluid are required. Culture and sensitivity testing of the blood or cerebrospinal fluid may be necessary in some cases of encephalitis to determine the cause and drugs of choice for treatment.

TREATMENT Antibiotics are used to treat bacterial infections. To reduce the brain swelling, corticosteroids and diuretics are used. The remaining treatment is directed at the symptoms and is mainly supportive care, which includes administration of intravenous fluids and pain relievers, expression of the bladder and the use of enemas if required, massage of paralyzed muscles, use of anticonvulsant drugs to control seizures, and either medications or the use of cold water baths and cool enemas to reduce high fever.

PROGNOSIS Many cases of encephalitis respond well to treatment, but the prognosis is always guarded in any disease or disorder involving the nervous system. Some recovered dogs are left with partial paralysis or epilepsy.

Meningitis

Meningitis is an inflammation or infection of the outer linings of the brain and spinal cord. The causes, symptoms, diagnosis, and treatments are similar to those of encephalitis, and the two diseases are often seen together. Specific diagnostic signs of meningitis are a rigid neck, refusal to lower the head, and obvious pain when the head or neck area are touched.

Brain Trauma or Injury

When a dog receives a severe head injury, it can cause one or more of the following effects:

Concussion. This is a violent jar or shock which shakes up the brain cells.

Contusion. This is a bruising of the brain tissue which occurs when the brain hits hard against the inner skull.

Laceration. This is a tearing of the brain tissue.

Compression. This is a pressing or squeezing of the brain from fractures of the skull, blood clots, abscesses, and hemorrhage.

Edema. This is a swelling of the brain cells with fluid, and occurs in nearly all cases of brain infections or trauma. Because the brain is enclosed in the rigid skull, it cannot expand to any extent before serious symptoms arise from the pressure on the brain tissue; without treatment, this can be fatal quickly.

Automobile accidents are the most frequent cause of brain injury in dogs. In puppies, a common cause is being stepped on or dropped.

SYMPTOMS Dogs that receive a severe head injury will be unconscious. If the injury is not traumatic enough to lead to unconsciousness, early signs of brain injury will include vomiting, diarrhea, weakness, paralysis, and convulsions that may progress to coma if there is hemorrhaging or swelling of the brain.

DIAGNOSIS Head injury cases are emergencies, particularly if the dog is unconscious, and immediate treatment will be started based on the clinical and neurological signs. Later diagnostic work will include laboratory blood tests and x-rays.

TREATMENT An unconscious dog should be placed on a board and taken immediately to a veterinary hospital. If there is heart or respiratory arrest, cardiopulmonary resuscitation measures can be taken (*see* Chapter 16, Emergency Care; Emergency Cases: Cardiopulmonary Resuscitation), but the dog owner should not delay seeking emergency care while doing this. The main aim of veterinary emergency treatment is to ensure that the dog's airway is not blocked and to reduce swelling of the brain with corticosteroids and diuretics, given intravenously. Treatment of shock will also be essential.

If there is a fracture of the skull, a penetrating injury, or evidence of hemorrhaging, surgery will be necessary. Unless absolutely essential to relieve pressure on the brain, surgery is delayed until the dog's vital signs are stabilized. Many fracture repairs can be postponed for three or four days, and this has the advantage of allowing the veterinarian to assess the degree of brain damage before proceeding with what could be an unnecessary surgery.

PROGNOSIS   The prognosis will depend on the severity of the brain injury, the speed with which treatment is given, and the amount of brain swelling. If the dog recovers consciousness early and there are no other serious injuries or evidence of nervous system damage, the prognosis is good. Unfortunately, some dogs recover consciousness quickly, only to relapse in a few hours due to slow hemorrhaging or edema, and in these cases the prognosis is more guarded. If the dog fails to recover consciousness within twenty-four hours the prognosis is poor. Some dogs will recover, but will be left partially paralyzed as a result of the injury, and in these cases, unless the paralysis is very severe, it is worth waiting a few months to see if the nervous system damage will repair itself.

DISEASES AND DISORDERS OF THE SPINAL CORD

Intervertebral (Spinal) Disc Disease (*See* Chapter 13, The Musculoskeletal System)

Spinal Cord Trauma or Injury

Since it is an extension of the brain, the spinal cord is susceptible to the effects of concussion, contusion, laceration, compression, or edema (*see* Brain Trauma or Injury, earlier in this chapter). Dogs are more prone to spinal cord injury than people because the dog's spinal cord nearly completely fills the spinal canal, and as a result there is not as much space available for swelling when an injury occurs. The most common causes of spinal cord injury in dogs are accidents, bullet wounds, fractures and dislocations, and intervertebral disc disease.

SYMPTOMS The signs of spinal cord injury depend on the area affected, the amount of displacement of the cord, and the degree of swelling and/or bleeding in the region of the injury. The most commonly affected area is between the thirteenth thoracic vertebra and the second lumbar vertebra—the lower back region behind the rib cage. Injury here results in rear leg and tail paralysis and loss of bowel and bladder function. There may also be signs of shock and other injuries.

DIAGNOSIS The diagnosis is made by the symptoms, a physical and neurological examination, laboratory blood and urine tests if shock is present, and x-rays.

TREATMENT A dog with a spinal cord injury should be moved with care on a flat board. Some may require sedation before moving because of aggressiveness caused by the pain; they should also be muzzled in such instances to prevent anyone from getting bitten.

The treatment is the same as for intervertebral disc disease (*see* Chapter 13, The Musculoskeletal System; Diseases and Disorders of the Skeletal System: Intervertebral (Spinal) Disc Disease), with the addition of treatment for shock and for any wounds or other injuries that may be present.

PROGNOSIS If sensation remains or returns to the paralyzed legs, the prognosis is much more favorable than if these areas continue to be insensitive.

Myelitis

Myelitis is an inflammation or infection of the spinal cord; it is often accompanied by meningitis. The causes are bacterial, fungal, or viral infections and trauma.

The diagnosis, symptoms, and treatments are the same as for spinal cord trauma, except that the dog may have a high fever if an infection is present. Antibiotics will be required if the infection is bacterial. Culture and sensitivity testing of the cerebrospinal fluid may also be required to determine the cause and drugs of choice for treatment.

DISEASES AND DISORDERS OF THE PERIPHERAL NERVES

The peripheral nervous system includes the twelve cranial nerves and the thirty-six or thirty-seven pairs of spinal nerves, which branch out to serve all other areas of the body. The

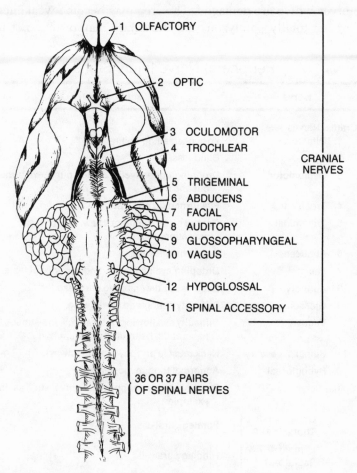

1 OLFACTORY

2 OPTIC

3 OCULOMOTOR
4 TROCHLEAR

CRANIAL
NERVES

5 TRIGEMINAL
6 ABDUCENS
7 FACIAL
8 AUDITORY
9 GLOSSOPHARYNGEAL
10 VAGUS

12 HYPOGLOSSAL

11 SPINAL ACCESSORY

36 OR 37 PAIRS
OF SPINAL NERVES

The Peripheral Nervous System (Underside of Brain)

most frequent cause of damage to the peripheral nerves is from injury due to accidents and dog fights. Other causes are tumors, infections, congenital defects, poisons, and certain vitamin and mineral deficiencies.

SYMPTOMS Injury to any of the peripheral nerves results in loss of motor (movement) and/or sensory function. The area supplied by the nerve can become paralyzed or lose all sensation, or both, depending on the function of the nerve or nerves which are damaged. The area may become weakened, but not totally paralyzed, and the injury may or may not be

Peripheral Nerve Injury Signs

Nerve	Signs of Injury
Cranial Nerves	
1. Olfactory	Loss of smelling ability.
2. Optic	Blindness.
3. Oculomotor	Drooping upper eyelid, dilated pupil, eye turned out and down.
4. Trochlear	Eye turned up and inward.
5. Trigeminal	Cannot close mouth or chew, loss of face sensation.
6. Abducens	Eye turned inward.
7. Facial	Drooping eyelid, mouth, and ear; loss of taste.
8. Auditory	Deafness and/or circling and head tilt.
9. Glossopharyngeal	Difficulty eating and swallowing.
10. Vagus	Difficulty swallowing. Also affects intestinal, pancreatic, heart, and lung function.
11. Spinal accessory	Neck muscle atrophy (wasting away).
12. Hypoglossal	Abnormal tongue movements.
Spinal Nerves	Paralysis of area supplied by nerve, such as, for example:
Cervical 5–8 & Thoracic 1–2	Foreleg paralysis.
Lumbar 4–7 & Sacral 1–3	Hindleg paralysis.

accompanied by pain. The preceding chart outlines briefly the major signs of injury to the peripheral nerves.

Nerves may also be injured in any area of the body, such as the radial nerve of the foreleg, or the tibial nerve of the hindleg. Specific signs of paralysis related to the areas these nerves supply will be evident and diagnostic.

DIAGNOSIS   Diagnosis is made by the symptoms, a physical and neurological examination, and x-rays.

TREATMENT   Medical treatment involves immobilizing the affected area if possible, and using anti-inflammatory agents, such as corticosteroids, to reduce swelling. Good nursing care and massage are also essential.

Surgical repair can be attempted, depending on the type of injury, location of the nerve, and the extent of the injury. If a limb or the tail is involved, and there is no response to medical or surgical treatment, then amputation may be necessary.

PROGNOSIS   As in all types of nervous system injury, it is worth waiting a few months to see if the damaged nerve regains its function before deciding on more complicated surgeries or euthanasia.

13

The Musculoskeletal System

The musculoskeletal system is made up of the following structures:

Muscle. Tissue consisting of elongated fibers that contract when stimulated by nerves to produce motion of the body.

Skeleton. The bony framework of the body.

Cartilage. Fibrous tissue composing most of the embryo skeleton, which later develops into bone. Cartilage also covers opposing bones in the joints.

Tendon. A fibrous cord by which a muscle is attached to a bone.

Ligament. A band of strong, fibrous tissue connecting two bones at a joint, serving to support and strengthen joints.

Bursa. A saclike cavity filled with a thick fluid and surrounded by a fibrous covering. Bursae serve to reduce friction and are found over bones and between tendons in areas where friction can occur.

Joint. The place of union of two or more bones of the skeleton, for example, the elbow.

DISEASES AND DISORDERS OF THE SKELETAL SYSTEM

Hip Dysplasia

Dysplasia means abnormal development. Simply defined, hip dysplasia is a looseness or instability of the ball-and-socket joint of the hip. In hip dysplasia the joint socket, or acetabulum, is too shallow, resulting in the head of the femur, (the leg bone) which is often too flat, slipping out of the socket. Eventually this leads to arthritic (inflammation of a joint) changes in the joint.

In dogs, the cause is unknown, although it does appear to be an inherited condition. While not present at birth, it can appear as early as six months of age. The exact mode of inheritance has not yet been fully determined. Large breeds, particularly German shepherds and Saint Bernards, are most frequently affected. Young dogs that grow rapidly or become overweight from being fed high-calorie diets have a higher incidence of this disorder.

SYMPTOMS The symptoms depend on the severity of the dysplasia and include some or all of the following:

- Lameness, particularly after vigorous or extended exercise.
- A swaying or wobbling gait (very apparent if the dog is seen walking away).
- Stiffness, particularly in the morning.
- Difficulty in, or reluctance to, standing up.
- Pain in the hip area, which can lead to limping.
- A change in temperament as a result of pain.
- Worsening of the condition in cold, damp weather.
- Poor development of the thigh and pelvic muscles.

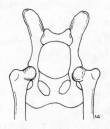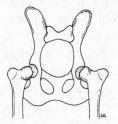

Normal Hip Joint/Hip Dysplasia

DIAGNOSIS The diagnosis is made by the history, symptoms, and a veterinary physical examination, and confirmed by x-rays of the hip joints. There is a grading system to describe the severity of the hip dysplasia visible on x-rays; Grade 1 is minimal evidence of hip dysplasia and Grade 4 is the most severe. The earliest a diagnosis can be made by x-rays is three to four months of age, and many cases do not show any evidence of hip dysplasia on x-ray until the dog is two years old and sometimes even older.

TREATMENT Although there is no cure, medical and/or surgical treatments are available and, in most cases, are effective. Treatment is only undertaken if the dog is in pain; many severely affected dogs have no pain because eventually a false hip joint forms.

Medical treatment involves the use of pain relievers, aspirin, and corticosteroid drugs. The dog should have warm, dry quarters, should not be allowed to get overweight, and should be limited in exercise to what it can handle without resulting stiffness or lameness.

Surgical treatments may be necessary if medical treatments are not effective or if the dog can no longer get around without severe discomfort. These treatments vary from cutting certain muscles and tendons to removal of the head of the femur and even to total hip replacement. Except in advanced cases, most dogs respond well to surgical treatment, but the improvement seldom lasts more than a few years.

PROGNOSIS Few dogs should have to be euthanized because of hip dysplasia since the response to treatments allows most affected dogs to live out their normal life span without total lameness setting in. Of course, affected dogs should never be used for breeding; neutering is advisable because of the hereditary nature of this problem.

PREVENTION Anyone buying a purebred dog from a breed that is commonly afflicted with hip dysplasia should request a certificate from the breeder that the line from which the puppy-of-choice is bred is not subject to this disease. The

Orthopedic Foundation for Animals (OFA), located at the University of Missouri, provides OFA certification to dogs shown by x-ray to be free of hip dysplasia at twenty-four months. The OFA maintains a registry of purebred dogs certified to be free of hip dysplasia, and it is well worth paying the extra cost the breeder will need to ask for a puppy whose parents are OFA-certified. The puppy itself cannot be certified, as hip dysplasia is seldom present in the young dog. Certification does not guarantee that a dog or its progeny will not develop hip dysplasia at some time in the future, but it reduces the odds considerably. It is also the only program presently available that attempts to eliminate this problem from affected breeds.

Other Congenital and Developmental Skeletal Deformities

There are numerous skeletal deformities in dogs, but most, fortunately, are rare. Some of those more commonly encountered are:

Hemivertebra is an abnormality in which one side of a vertebra is incompletely developed. Depending on the severity it may produce spinal curvature or arching. Most cases do not lead to clinical signs, but severe abnormalities lead to paralysis. Surgical treatment is possible, although it is seldom done. Hemivertebrae in the tail region result in a kinked or screw tail.

Spina bifida is an abnormality in which the bony enclosure of the spinal cord is defective, sometimes resulting in protrusion of the spinal cord. While severe cases lead to paralysis, Spina bifida may be present without causing any problems. Surgical treatment is possible.

Absence of ribs is an uncommon abnormality, except for the 13th rib. This seldom causes problems, but can lead to some spinal curvature.

Elbow dysplasia is a failure of part of the ulna bone to fuse during development; also called *ununited anconeal pro-*

cess. This condition leads to foreleg lameness. It can be treated by removing the loose bone or anchoring it to the ulna surgically.

Epiphyseal dysplasia is an abnormality in the growth centers of the bones. Treatment is not usually necessary, although affected dogs do not reach normal size.

Osteochondrosis is a disorder resulting in excessive cartilage formation. This condition leads to lameness. Treatment involves restricted exercise and corticosteroids for mild cases and surgical intervention for severe cases.

Legg-Perthes disease is the destruction of the head of the femur from a lack of blood supply. This disease leads to hindleg lameness. Some dogs recover with rest and corticosteroids, but most require surgery.

Dwarfism is underdevelopment of the body. There are a number of different causes of dwarfism, and some respond to replacement hormone treatment.

Bone Infections (Osteomyelitis)

Although many people do not realize it, bone is living tissue that can become infected; fortunately it can also repair itself, particularly with the aid of modern medicine. Infection of the bone is called osteomyelitis and can be acute or chronic. Acute infections show up quickly, while those that are chronic spread slowly and symptoms can take months to develop.

The most common causes of bone infections in both people and dogs are staphylococcal bacteria, followed by streptococcal bacteria, and, more rarely, other bacterial and fungal organisms. Bone infections can arise from infections in other areas of the body carried to the bone by the bloodstream. The more common causes of bone infections in dogs are from outside the body via bite wounds, other puncture wounds, compound fractures, and bone surgeries. Severe dental disease can lead to infection of the bones of the jaws.

SYMPTOMS   The initial signs are pain, swelling, fever, and

if a limb is involved, lameness. These signs are usually accompanied by depression and loss of appetite. In time the infection usually breaks through the skin, and a blood-tinged or pus discharge occurs.

DIAGNOSIS   The diagnosis is made by the history and clinical signs, confirmed by blood tests and x-rays. It is advisable to have the discharge cultured in order to identify the organism that is causing the infection and also to run a sensitivity test to determine which antibiotic will be effective in treatment. Although these tests are extra costs, bone infections can be difficult to clear up and a hit-or-miss use of antibiotics can make the condition worse.

TREATMENT   In most cases it will be necessary to drain the wound surgically and remove all dead and infected tissue from the bone. Vigorous and often long-term antibiotic treatment will be essential, both systemically (by injection or mouth) and locally (into the wound). The wound will either be left open or closed with a tube inserted for drainage. Although most bone infections clear up with adequate treatment, some do not respond and require more extensive surgery and long-term treatment.

Arthritis

Arthritis is an inflammation of the joints; it occurs in dogs as well as people, in a very similar way in both. There are many different types of arthritis, and the term "rheumatism" is used as a general classification for all diseases of the joints. There are three main types of arthritis in dogs.

Septic arthritis, caused by a bacterial infection of the joint, most commonly arises from a puncture wound into the joint or from an infection elsewhere in the body that is carried to the joint via the bloodstream.

Osteoarthritis is caused by degenerative disease of the joints associated with age, from acute trauma to the joints by accidents, or from chronic trauma occurring, for example, with the dislocation that occurs in hip dysplasia.

Rheumatoid arthritis is similar to, but not quite the same as, the disease of the same name in humans. The cause has not been fully determined.

DIAGNOSIS   All these diseases are diagnosed in dogs by the history, clinical signs, a veterinary physical examination, and confirmed by x-rays.

SYMPTOMS   *Septic arthritis,* from bacteria entering a joint, leads to a red, hot, swollen, and painful joint, which frequently discharges fluid or pus. It may be accompanied by fever, depression, and if in a limb joint, lameness.

Osteoarthritis from aging or trauma leads to degenerative changes in the joints, particularly on the surfaces of the bones (cartilage) in the joints. It causes pain and stiffness, and its development and progression are slow. Except when the cause is trauma, dogs are usually over eight years old before signs occur.

Rheumatoid arthritis occurs more often in two- to five-year-old dogs of the larger breeds. The first sign is usually lameness, but no obvious swelling or redness is seen in the early stages. Later the affected joints enlarge. Sometimes the disease will go into remission and then recur.

TREATMENT   *Septic arthritis* requires immediate treatment with antibiotics, and the joint may require surgical drainage and the use of antibiotics locally or injected into the joint. Even with prompt and effective treatment, some joint damage will remain.

Osteoarthritis treatment involves the use of aspirin, or cortiscosteroids if aspirin is ineffective, a warm environment, massage, heating pads, and sometimes injections into the affected joints.

Rheumatoid arthritis treatment is similar to that for osteoarthritis.

Intervertebral (Spinal) Disc Disease

Intervertebral discs are found between each two vertebrae (bones of the spinal column); they are designed to absorb

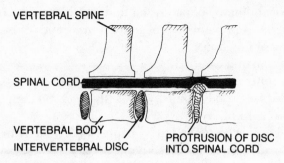

VERTEBRAL SPINE

SPINAL CORD

VERTEBRAL BODY
INTERVERTEBRAL DISC

PROTRUSION OF DISC
INTO SPINAL CORD

Intervertebral (Spinal) Disc Disease

shock and allow movement of the spine. Each disc has an inner soft nucleus and an outer fibrous capsule. With age and disease the discs dehydrate and lose elasticity and can, as a result, rupture or protrude into the spinal cord where they cause pain and loss of function. Certain breeds of dogs, as discussed later, are more susceptible to intervertebral disc disease.

SYMPTOMS   The symptoms depend on which area of the spinal cord is affected and on the extent of compression of the cord. Protrusion in the neck region results in a stiff neck, pain, and sometimes front leg lameness. Protrusion in the lower spinal column regions causes rear leg lameness or paralysis, not as much pain as in the neck region, and sometimes loss of bladder control and retention of feces.

DIAGNOSIS   The diagnosis is made from the history, symptoms, a physical and neurological examination, and x-rays.

TREATMENT   Treatment is medical or surgical, depending on the degree of paralysis.

Medical treatment. Some or all of the following approaches may be used in medical treatment:

1. Administration of anti-inflammatory agents, such as corticosteroids, to reduce the swelling.
2. Enforced rest or confinement.

3. Physical therapy of paralyzed limbs with massage and manipulations to prevent loss of muscle mass and assist in the regaining of function.

4. Good nursing care.

5. Pain relievers, used cautiously; if the pain is masked too much, dogs tend to become overly active and can then worsen the spinal cord injury.

6. The bladder may need to be expressed manually or catheterized, and enemas may also be necessary, if these areas are paralyzed.

Surgical Treatment. There are a number of surgical techniques to relieve the compression on the spinal cord, and one of these may be recommended if the paralysis is severe and the x-rays and other diagnostic tests indicate that the surgical approach could have a favorable outcome.

Some dogs do not recover the use of their rear legs. A special cart has been designed to support the paralyzed rear legs of dogs that cannot be helped by other treatments. It allows the dog to move about and is surprisingly well accepted by most dogs.

PROGNOSIS The immediate prognosis is poor if there is no sensation in the paralyzed rear legs. The long-term prognosis is also poor if there is no improvement after two months, especially after surgery.

SUSCEPTIBILITY Unfortunately, intervertebral disc disease is a relatively common problem in dogs, particularly in the chondrodystrophic breeds. Chondrodystrophy is a type of dwarfism in which there is thickening of the joint regions; short, bowed legs; a disproportion of the body and limbs; and spinal cord abnormalities. This type of body structure places additional stress on the spinal column and often results in disc protrusions. The condition is both inherited and congenital, and is characteristic of the following breeds of dogs: dachshund, English bulldog, Pekingese, French bulldog, pug,

American cocker spaniel, King Charles spaniel, bassett hound, beagle, boxer, and bull mastiff.

The dachshund is the breed most affected, with the risk of occurrence ten times greater than for all other breeds combined. The disease occurs in about 20% of the breed. The peak incidence is from three to six years of age. While dachshunds are genetically predisposed to disc disease, it does not follow any simple pattern of hereditary transmission. However, litters of affected dogs or affected lines do have a higher incidence of the disease.

In choosing a puppy, whether a dachshund or any of the breeds susceptible to spinal disc disease, it is advisable to check the breeding line for disc problems by asking the breeder to show the potential buyer *older* close relatives. (The parents of the litter may be too young to show any signs of disc problems yet.) If the relatives are not at the kennel, a buyer should ask for the names and phone numbers of the owners of at least three of the dogs which are closely related to the puppy-of-choice.

Chondrodystrophic breeds of dogs have an abnormal skeletal system and are deliberately bred to propagate these abnormalities as characteristic of each of these breeds. These abnormalities frequently lead to skeletal problems, not only in the spinal cord, but in the limbs and other areas of the body. For those dog owners who like these breeds, there is a risk of disc problems developing when the dog matures. However, since all breeds of dogs have their own individual hereditary health risks, this should not unduly influence anyone who particularly likes these breeds.

Fractures

A fracture is a break or rupture in a bone. Fractures in dogs are caused by trauma or injury to the body, most commonly due to automobile accidents, falls, or fighting. There are many medical terms used to describe fractures, some of which are:

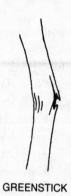

GREENSTICK

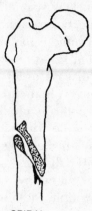

SPIRAL

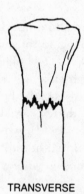

TRANSVERSE

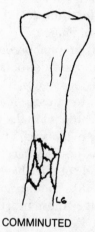

COMMINUTED

Common Fractures

- *Simple, or closed, fracture,* which occurs if there is no wound to the outside skin.
- *Compound fracture,* which occurs if the broken bone breaks through the skin.
- *Greenstick fracture,* a condition in which one side of the bone is broken and the other is bent.
- *Comminuted fracture,* in which the bone is splintered or crushed.
- *Transverse fracture,* in which there is a break across the bone.
- *Impacted fracture,* in which one fragment of bone is driven firmly into another.
- *Spiral fracture,* in which the bones have been twisted apart.
- *Avulsion fracture,* in which there is a tearing away of part of the bone.

SYMPTOMS The signs of a fracture are obvious in most cases. The bones may be seen protruding through the skin, or if it is a closed fracture, signs of swelling, pain, and inability to move the area affected will be evident. Signs of shock may also accompany a fracture, and there may be other more serious injuries.

DIAGNOSIS The diagnosis is made by the symptoms and a physical examination, and confirmed by x-rays.

TREATMENT Taking care to avoid a bite, a dog owner should try to restrain a dog with a fracture, and if possible, to muzzle the injured dog before attempting to handle it. If a spinal fracture is suspected, the dog should be placed on a board and taken immediately to a veterinarian for treatment. If a limb is fractured, the limb should be supported gently on a pillow or a towel and the dog taken to a veterinarian. If the fracture area is bleeding, a pressure pad or cloth should be used to control the bleeding (*see* Chapter 18, Home Medical Care; Home Treatments: Bleeding). If the bone is protruding

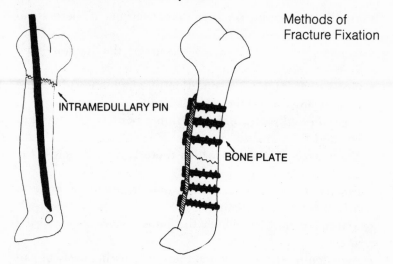

Methods of
Fracture Fixation

INTRAMEDULLARY PIN

BONE PLATE

through the skin, the wound should be covered with a sterile pad or a clean cloth.

In limb fractures a splint can be made out of cardboard or newspapers taped around the leg before transporting the dog to a veterinary hospital (*see* Chapter 18, Home Medical Care; Home Treatments: Splints). It is best to seek immediate veterinary care in most fracture cases, rather than spend time trying to apply a splint, as many of these dogs are suffering from shock or more serious injuries than the obvious fracture, and require emergency treatment. Few fractures need immediate repair, but the accompanying injuries or shock seen in most fracture cases in dogs are real emergencies.

The approach to repairing a fracture depends to a considerable degree on the type of fracture and the amount of damage to the adjacent tissues. Medically there are four main therapies which must be applied in all fractures.

1. *Reduction,* which involves correcting any displacement that has occurred in the bone alignment by placing the broken ends together (also called setting a bone). Reduction is done externally by manipulation in closed uncomplicated fractures,

and the alignment is checked by x-rays. In compound or complicated fractures, the reduction is done internally during surgical repair.

2. *Fixation*, which involves fastening the broken fragments together. External fixation is done by using a cast or splint after the fracture has been reduced. Internal fixation is done surgically using wires, metal pins, metal plates, or lag screws to fasten the broken bone fragments together. Some of these surgical fixation devices are left in the bone permanently.

3. *Immobilization*, which is done internally, externally, or both to keep the break from moving as it heals. Internal fixation by surgical means is one form of immobilization. External casts or splints are other methods of immobilization.

4. *Restoration of function*, which involves massage and therapy. Bone is living tissue and can repair itself if the gap between the bone fracture lines is not too great, and if movement is limited during the healing process. Bone heals more slowly than other body tissues, and most fractures need a minimum of six weeks to heal. Unfortunately, during this period the function of the muscles, tendons, and joints in the affected area deteriorates, so after healing is complete it is important to slowly restore these functions with massage and graduated exercise.

PROGNOSIS   While most fractures heal well, some do not. This is a more common problem in dogs than in people, since it is difficult to keep the fracture area immobilized in a dog. Dogs often rip off the cast or splint, or reinjure the area. In these instances, further surgery may be required.

If there is a lot of tissue damage or if the bone is fractured beyond repair in a limb or the tail, amputation may be the only alternative.

COST AND CHOICE OF METHOD FOR FRACTURE REPAIR
Veterinarians do take into account the cost of fracture repair to the dog owner, and wherever possible they offer alternative approaches to treatment, together with estimated charges. In

serious fractures, the surgical approach offers the best prognosis for full recovery of function, but the use of a cast or splint is less costly. Many clients choose the less costly treatment and very often the outcome is excellent; if this fails, the client will then have the added expense of surgery and a poorer prognosis because of the delay. The body, human or animal, has remarkable powers of healing, and some very serious fractures heal beautifully with no treatment at all. However, this is not a risk worth taking because some dreadful deformities result from fractures that are not taken care of, and it is difficult for veterinarians to predict which will heal naturally and which will not.

Dislocations

A dislocation occurs when a bone is forced out of place at a joint. The cause is from trauma or injury and often involves a twisting motion. The dislocation may be partial or complete.

SYMPTOMS   In dislocations, the joint will usually look out of shape and will be painful and swollen.

DIAGNOSIS   Diagnosis is made by the symptoms and a physical examination, and confirmed by x-rays.

TREATMENT   An anesthetic will be required while the dislocated joint is manipulated back into place. Occasionally surgery will be required to replace the dislocated joint. Sometimes a cast or splint will be applied if there has been severe injury to the joint. Pain relievers, rest, and restricted exercise will be necessary for only a few days in uncomplicated cases.

PROGNOSIS   Most dogs recover without complication, but some will have recurrent dislocations of a particular joint and in these cases, surgical repair will be necessary.

Kneecap Dislocation (Patellar Luxation)

Partial or complete dislocation of the small bone in front of the knee, called the patella, or kneecap, is not an uncommon problem in small dogs.

In many of these breeds, such as Pomeranians, Yorkshire terriers, Chihuahuas, and miniature and toy poodles, it appears to be due to a hereditary structural defect of the knee joint. It is ten times more common in these breeds than in other dogs, and is usually first seen about five to six months of age. However, the kneecap can be dislocated in any dog from trauma or injury.

SYMPTOMS   When the kneecap dislocates, there is usually not much pain, but the dog will carry the leg off the ground. In severe cases or those in which both kneecaps are involved, lameness will result.

DIAGNOSIS   Diagnosis is made from the symptoms and a veterinary physical examination in which the dislocated kneecap is palpated, and confirmed by x-rays.

TREATMENT   The dislocated kneecap can be replaced while the dog is sedated, but in recurrent cases, surgery will be necessary to reinforce the knee joint and prevent the patella from dislocating again.

PREVENTION   Because kneecap dislocation appears to be a hereditary problem in certain small breeds of dogs, anyone purchasing one of these breeds should ask the breeder if any of the dogs related to the puppy-of-choice has this problem. It is also a good precaution to have the puppy examined by a veterinarian before the final purchase, as quite often the abnormality in the knee joint can be recognized by palpation and x-rays.

Ligament Rupture

Ligaments are bands of strong fibrous tissue connecting two bones at a joint. They rupture as a result of a severe trauma or injury. In dogs, the cruciate ligaments in the knee joint are frequently ruptured in accidents; however, ligament rupture may also occur as a result of disease in a joint unrelated to trauma.

SYMPTOMS   If a ligament is ruptured, the affected joint cannot function normally. If the knee joint is involved, there is lameness and the joint can slide back and forth beyond the normal range of motion. Most ligament ruptures occur from trauma and are accompanied by other injuries in the area, so pain, swelling, and tenderness are often also seen.

DIAGNOSIS The diagnosis is made from the symptoms, a physical examination, and in some cases, x-rays.

TREATMENT Ligament ruptures need to be repaired surgically as soon as possible after the injury for full recovery of joint function. Provided that the joint damage is not too severe, surgical repair will be successful.

Sprain

A sprain is similar to a ligament rupture, except that the ligament is torn, but not completely ruptured. The cause, symptoms, and diagnosis, while less severe, are similar to rupture.

Treatment involves the use of cold compresses and support bandages to restrict movement, until healing is complete.

DISEASES AND DISORDERS OF THE MUSCULAR SYSTEM

Muscle Atrophy

Atrophy means a wasting away or a reduction in size. Muscle atrophy refers most commonly to the reduction in size of a muscle but not of the number of muscle fibers, although some diseases do destroy the muscle fibers as well. There are many causes, but for clarity of description, muscle atrophy is broken down into three main categories:

1. Atrophy from not using the muscle. This is due primarily to prolonged inactivity. The most common incidence of this is when a leg is in a cast or splint, or is injured and not used for weight-bearing by the animal. In most cases, these types of atrophy are reversible if the muscle is again put into use.

2. Atrophy due to damage to the nerves supplying the muscle. Muscles cannot contract without nerve transmission stimuli. The injury can be in the spinal cord or the nerves leading to or within the muscle; the nerves may be damaged by diseases that affect nerve transmissions. Some of these causes are reversible with time or treatment, but many are not, and severe muscle atrophy results.

3. Atrophy from disease of the muscle itself. The more frequent causes of this are bacterial infections from a wound, muscle degeneration diseases, tumors, and bleeding into the muscle. Some of these respond to treatment; others are progressive despite the best medical care.

Bursitis

Bursae are saclike cavities filled with a thick fluid and surrounded by a fibrous covering; they serve to reduce friction between tendons and over bones. There are two types of bursae: true bursae, which are present at birth and are found between bone and tendon; and false bursae, called hygromas, which develop as a result of trauma and are found over bony prominences under the skin. The condition is called bursitis when either of these types of bursae becomes inflamed or infected.

The cause of bursitis is trauma or injury, which may be complicated by bacterial infection. Hygromas are seen mostly over the elbow area in large breeds of dogs and are caused by mild, continual trauma to this area from the weight of the dog, usually as a result of lying on hard surfaces.

SYMPTOMS There may be local swelling and pain, particularly after exercise, in the area of the affected bursa. Hygromas are readily visible and are seen most often in the elbow area, but may occur over any bony prominence. Initially, they are small, soft swellings, but in time they can become large and hard. Sometimes hygromas and bursae become infected, rupture, and drain.

DIAGNOSIS The diagnosis of bursitis is made by the symptoms and a physical examination; and in the case of hygromas, by observation. If infection is present, a culture and sensitivity test of the discharge may be needed to identify the bacteria and determine the most effective antibiotic for treatment.

TREATMENT True bursitis usually responds to rest. Some cases require anti-inflammatory drugs such as corticosteroids to reduce the swelling and pain. Antibiotics will be required if infection is present.

Hygromas are more difficult to treat, but fortunately most can be left alone, unless they are causing pain, increasing in size, or are infected. Small hygromas respond well to surgical drainage, but larger ones may require surgical removal. Unfortunately, hygromas tend to recur in heavy dogs, and wound healing is often a problem after surgical removal because of the continuing trauma to the area from the weight of the dog. Good nursing care is essential. Soft bedding and weight reduction, if the dog is overweight, are helpful preventives.

Myositis

Myositis is an inflammation or infection of a muscle. The most common cause of myositis in dogs is from penetrating wounds into the muscle. It can also occur from extension of an infection from other nearby tissues, such as a bone infection. Occasionally it is caused by an intramuscular injection.

SYMPTOMS Myositis causes pain and swelling of the muscle. If a limb is involved, there is usually lameness. The infection may break through the skin and discharge pus.

DIAGNOSIS The diagnosis is made by the symptoms and a physical examination. X-rays may be needed to make sure there is not a foreign body in the muscle that is causing the infection.

TREATMENT Treatment involves the use of antibiotics. Some cases will require surgical opening and draining of the infected muscle.

Strain

A strain is an injury to a muscle or tendon, caused by overstretching or pulling a muscle, most commonly as a result of overexertion.

SYMPTOMS A strain causes pain and stiffness of the affected muscle.

DIAGNOSIS The diagnosis is made by the symptoms and a physical examination.

TREATMENT Most strains repair themselves with rest, the use of a heating pad to relieve the pain, and gentle massage.

Tendinitis and Tendon Rupture

A tendon is a fibrous cord by which a muscle is attached to a bone. These tendons can rupture or become inflamed (tendinitis). Trauma or injury is the most common cause of both tendinitis and rupture of a tendon.

SYMPTOMS The symptoms are pain and stiffness of the affected muscle. If the tendon is ruptured, the muscle cannot function properly.

DIAGNOSIS The diagnosis is made by the symptoms and a physical examination. Identification of such injuries can be difficult in dogs.

TREATMENT Tendinitis usually responds to rest, pain relievers, and restricted exercise of the affected area. Sometimes corticosteroids are used in treatment. If the injury becomes chronic or the tendon is ruptured, surgical repair will be necessary.

NUTRITIONAL DISEASES AND DISORDERS OF THE MUSCULOSKELETAL SYSTEM
(*See also* Chapter 1, Nutrition.)

Nutritional deficiencies and, less commonly, excesses, can lead to many bone and muscle diseases and disorders in dogs.

Fortunately, with the easy availability of nutritionally complete and balanced dog foods these problems are not frequently encountered in dogs today. Some nutrition-related problems of the musculoskeletal system occurring in dogs follow.

Calcium, Phophorus, and Vitamin D

Vitamin D, calcium, and phosphorus are interrelated, and deficiencies or imbalances can lead to bone disorders. A calcium and phosphorus imbalance, most usually low calcium and high phosphorus from an all-meat diet, can lead to poor growth, lameness, and soft bones. Phosphorus and/or vitamin D deficiency causes rickets in young dogs; the result is abnormal curvature of the long bones and thickening of the joints. In adults, rickets does not develop, but a similar condition called osteomalacia occurs and results in softening of the bones and lameness.

Excess vitamin D causes deposits of calcium in the soft tissues.

Copper

Deficiency: Severe bone changes, with curvature and shortening of the long bones and enlarged joints.

Magnesium

Deficiency: Muscle incoordination, weakness, and stiffness.

Excess: Suppresses bone growth.

Manganese

Excess: A condition similar to rickets occurs.

Lead

Excess: Lead lines can be seen in the bones on x-ray.

Zinc

Deficiency: Reduction in bone growth and muscle development.

Vitamin A

Deficiency: Growth stunted and bones fragile.
Excess: Bone development abnormalities.

Vitamin C

Deficiency: This is very unusual because dogs can synthesize their own vitamin C. A few dogs have a defect in this metabolism, and lameness and swelling of the joints results.

Vitamin E and Selenium

Deficiency: Stunted growth.

Protein

Deficiency: Stunted growth.

Overnutrition

Skeletal problems, particularly in young dogs, can be caused by overnutrition.

14

Infectious, Respiratory, and Hormonal Diseases

LABORATORY TESTS FOR DISEASE DIAGNOSIS

By and large, the laboratory tests done on pets today are the same as those done on people. They are required to diagnose disease accurately, or to monitor the progress of the pet during treatment. The costs of these tests are related to the high cost of the sophisticated equipment and the use of trained technologists to perform many of these tests. In-house laboratory charges are usually lower than those of outside commercial laboratories, but not all veterinary hospitals have their own laboratory facilities. Many use outside commercial laboratories and pass the charges on to the dog owner.

A course of treatment based on a misdiagnosis is useless and expensive and may cost the pet its life because of the delay. Laboratory tests aid in reaching an accurate diagnosis, which is essential for effective treatment; conversely, should they show that the disease cannot be treated or is terminal, unnecessary treatments and suffering by the pet can be avoided.

Following are some of the laboratory tests performed by veterinarians.

Blood examination. Microscopic examination of red blood cells, white blood cells, and platelets aids in the diagnosis

236

and treatment of anemias, infections, allergies, leukemias, bleeding disorders, and blood parasites.

Urinalysis. Gross and microscopic examination of urine aids in the diagnosis and treatment of kidney and urinary tract diseases, diabetes, and heart and liver diseases.

Tests for parasites. Fecal examinations detect intestinal parasites. Skin scrapings detect mites which cause mange and the fungus infection that causes ringworm. Blood examinations are used to identify heartworms.

Body fluid tests. Blood and serum chemistries are measured to diagnose and monitor treatment in diseases of the kidneys, liver, pancreas, heart muscle, and thyroid gland. Cerebrospinal fluid is tested in brain and spinal cord injuries.

Bacteriological and fungal tests. Tests are performed on body fluids and discharges to determine which bacteria or fungi are causing disease. The bacterial and fungal organisms are grown on a special culture medium and are then identified. The bacteria are further tested against various antibiotics to determine which antibiotic will be effective in treatment; this is called sensitivity testing.

Hormone assays. Diseases of hormone-secreting glands, such as the thyroid, adrenal, ovaries, and testes, require hormonal assays for diagnosis and for monitoring treatment.

Cytology. Microscopic examination of tissue, also referred to as a biopsy, is used to diagnose benign and malignant tumors, as well as the type of damage to many body tissues and organs from infection and degenerative diseases.

VACCINATIONS

Vaccinations for dogs are vital and are not just a way for veterinarians to make money, as some pet owners suggest. As a matter of fact, veterinarians made a lot more money from infectious canine diseases before vaccines were developed. One of the reasons so many dogs live to a ripe old age these days is that vaccines are now available to protect them from many previously fatal infectious diseases.

Immunity

An animal's response to the invasion by an infectious organism, such as a bacterium or virus, is to develop antibodies against it in an attempt to fight off the invader. This is known as an immunologic response or the development of immunity. An animal can become immune to a disease either by having been exposed to it or by vaccination. In vaccination a harmless form of the disease organism is introduced into the body; this stimulates the body to produce antibodies against the disease, thus making the animal immune to it. A young puppy requires frequent vaccinations to build up immunity, and older dogs require periodic booster vaccinations to keep up their level of immunity.

During the first few days of life, a puppy receives a degree of immunity to some canine diseases through the colostrum of its mother's milk; this is one reason why it is most important to have a puppy nurse from its mother in the first few days of life. The immunity passed from the mother to the puppy is only for those diseases the mother has been exposed to and recovered from, or received vaccination against. The puppy is protected from these diseases for anywhere from four to twelve weeks. This maternal immunity passed to the puppy can interfere with a vaccination's effectiveness and it is difficult to determine when this immunity is depleted, which is another reason puppies need to be vaccinated early and given a number of doses.

Occasional adverse effects result from vaccinations, but this is rare, and overall, the benefits far outweigh the risks. Any older veterinarian can tell you that the chances of puppies surviving to adulthood were not good before the development of canine vaccines, and if they did make it, the pups were like children before human vaccines were developed, fighting off one infectious disease after another.

INFECTIOUS DISEASES FOR WHICH VACCINES ARE AVAILABLE

There are vaccines available now for eight infectious canine diseases, and continuing research may increase this number in the future. A description of each disease for which a vaccine is produced follows; they are not described in detail because they are seldom encountered by the conscientious dog owner today.

Canine Distemper is the most common viral infectious disease of dogs. This virus is highly contagious and invades all body tissues. It causes a generalized infection with respiratory, intestinal, and nervous system symptoms; it is fatal about 50% of the time, and recovered dogs may be left with nervous system disorders.

CANINE DISTEMPER AND MULTIPLE SCLEROSIS During the past few years, the media have brought to the public's attention the possibility of a relationship between canine distemper and multiple sclerosis. A great deal of research has been done on this subject, and the most recent studies concluded that canine distemper virus is not implicated as a cause of multiple sclerosis.

The background on this controversy began in 1975 when an outbreak of canine distemper occurred in the Faroe Islands at the same time as an epidemic of multiple sclerosis. When the blood of the human patients was tested for antibody titer (immunity level) to canine distemper virus, the titers in many were high. At the time it was thought that there was some connection between these two diseases. It was later found, however, that those tests had actually measured human measles virus antibodies and not canine distemper antibodies; the confusion arose because the human measles virus and the canine distemper virus are closely related. Further testing showed that the measles virus antibody is present in many adults, but is not related to multiple sclerosis. It has also been determined that measles in humans is not caused by canine distemper virus; it just happens that these closely related viruses respond similarly when tested, making it extremely difficult to distinguish between them in blood tests.

Infectious Canine Hepatitis is a viral disease caused by canine adenovirus type 1; it affects the liver, intestinal tract, and eyes. Many cases are fatal; occasionally a mild form occurs, leaving the dog with a blue cloudy appearance to the eyes.

A related virus, canine adenovirus type 2, causes a respiratory disease in dogs and is involved in the kennel cough disease complex, which as the name suggests results in a distressing chronic cough, that can last for months. The type 1 or type 2 virus vaccine provides protection against both viruses.

Canine Leptospirosis is a disease of dogs caused by a bacterial organism called a spirochete, which is spread via infected urine. Rats are the most common source of infection for dogs. The disease primarily affects the liver, gastrointestinal tract, and kidneys, and can lead to death from kidney failure.

Canine Parainfluenza is a viral respiratory infection. It is usually mild, but can be severe if other respiratory infectious organisms are also involved. It is highly contagious, especially where dogs are housed together, and is usually part of the kennel cough disease complex.

Canine Bordetellosis is a common bacterium in the respiratory tract of dogs. It is one of the causes of the kennel cough disease complex. It is also prevalent where dogs are housed together. In itself it is not a serious disease, but if other respiratory infections are present or complications occur, it can lead to pneumonia.

Canine Coronavirus is a highly contagious disease that causes loss of appetite, depression, and a sudden onset of vomiting and diarrhea. The virus was first identified in 1971, and a vaccine has recently become available. The symptoms are similar to canine parvovirus infection, although the disease is not as severe in puppies. The outcome of infection depends on the dog's age and condition.

Canine Parvovirus (CPV) is an infection caused by a virus related to the feline panleukopenia (distemper) virus. Cats with distemper do not infect dogs, however, although the viruses are close relatives. The parvovirus causes intestinal problems in dogs and can damage the heart in puppies. While it is not usually serious in adults, it can quickly be fatal in puppies.

CPV is a totally new disease in dogs, not a previously unrecognized disease. It was first recognized as a new disease in dogs in 1978 and quickly became a problem worldwide. Feline panleukopenia (FPL), previously called feline distemper, is also caused by a parvovirus. The origin of CPV is not really known, but experts researching this subject agree that CPV may have come from the FPL virus by mutation, or possibly CPV is a variant of the FPL virus. Whatever the origin, the virus adapted to dogs and rapid transmission occurred. However, cats with FPL do not directly infect dogs with CPV, as each of these parvoviruses is species-specific.

Infection in dogs depends on the age and health of the dog and the size of the infecting virus dose. Most adult dogs have no sign of the disease although they are infected and develop immunity. The most common symptom is diarrhea, followed by depression, vomiting, and loss of appetite. Adult dogs usually recover, particularly if given supportive veterinary treatment to prevent dehydration. Puppies younger than twelve weeks of age become seriously ill with bloody diarrhea and a high fever; even with treatment, few survive. A second form of the disease occurs in puppies and causes inflammation of the heart muscle, which rapidly proves fatal in most instances.

Rabies is a viral disease that can affect any warm-blooded mammal. The virus is present in the saliva of an infected animal and enters the body through any break in the skin or mucous membranes, and by inhaling airborne virus in caves heavily populated with infected bats. Skunks and bats are the most dangerous reservoirs of rabies. The disease affects the nervous system and is fatal once symptoms occur. Vaccination is mandatory in all areas of the United States and Canada.

Treatment

All of these diseases, except rabies, can be treated. Because most are viral there is no specific drug for treatment, but symptomatic and supportive veterinary care can save many dogs, even those with the more serious diseases. Antibiotics are used if the infection is bacterial or if secondary bacterial infection is complicating the case. Treatment can be prolonged and expensive, so preventive vaccination is always recommended to all dog owners by veterinarians. Nothing is quite as sad for a devoted dog owner as losing an older dog to one of these diseases, simply because the owner forgot to get a booster vaccination.

Vaccination Schedule

There is no rigid vaccination schedule for dogs, and dog owners should check with a local veterinary hospital for advice. Many factors influence the choice of a vaccination schedule, including the prevalence of the disease in the area, the general condition of the puppy or dog, the presence of parasites or other diseases, the age, and the type of vaccine. The following schedule may be used as a guideline.

While this vaccination schedule may seem like an awful lot of injections for a new puppy to endure, as many as five of these vaccines can be combined in one injection. And since not all vaccinations are needed in all areas, in reality only four or five injections are required in the first four months of a puppy's life to give it full protection. All these vaccines are available individually or in various combinations. The combination vaccines are just as effective as the individual vaccines, and are a lot easier on the puppy or dog and on the owner's pocketbook and schedule.

Canine Vaccination Schedule

Disease	Age First Vaccine (weeks)	Age Second Vaccine (weeks)	Age Third Vaccine (weeks)	Revaccin- ation Intervals (months)
Distemper	6–8	10–12	14–16	12
Infectious Canine Hepatitis	6–8	10–12	14–16	12
Parvovirus	6–8	10–12	14–16	12
Bordetellosis	6–8	10–12	14–16	12
Coronavirus	6–8	10–12	14–16	12
Parainfluenza	6–8	10–12	14–16	12
Leptospirosis	10–12	14–16	—	12
Rabies—Live Vaccine	12–16	—	—	12 or 36*
Rabies—Inactive Vaccine	12–16	—	—	12

* Revaccination interval depends on type of vaccine used.

INFECTIOUS DISEASES FOR WHICH NO VACCINES ARE AVAILABLE

Infectious diseases for which no vaccines are available are not encountered nearly as frequently as those infectious diseases for which vaccines are available. Experimental vaccines have been developed for some of these diseases, but because of the low incidence, the vaccines are not approved for routine use in dogs. The following chart outlines the causative agents for these diseases, the symptoms, and the treatment.

Other Infectious Diseases of Dogs

Cause	Symptoms/Prognosis	Treatment
Herpesvirus (virus)	Puppies: Diarrhea, respiratory signs. Usually fatal. Adults: Mild respiratory signs. Most recover.	Supportive and symptomatic.
Pseudorabies (virus)	Itching, convulsions, coma. Most die.	Supportive and symptomatic.
Brucellosis (bacteria)	Female: Abortion, vaginal discharge. Male: Testicle and prostate disease. Seldom fatal. May become chronic.	Antibiotics. Do not use for breeding.
Tetanus (bacteria)	Muscle spasms, lockjaw. Often fatal. (Can vaccinate if there is exposure risk.)	Antitoxin. Antibiotics. Supportive and symptomatic.
Anthrax (bacteria)	Rare. Depression, fever, swelling of face and throat. Often fatal.	Antibiotics. Supportive and symptomatic. Human hazard, so usually not treated.
Tuberculosis (bacteria)	Rare. Loss of weight, coughing.	Human hazard, so usually not treated.
Tularemia (bacteria)	Skin abscesses, chills, eye discharge. Most adults recover.	Antibiotics. Supportive and symptomatic.
Listeriosis (bacteria)	Rare. Respiratory and nervous system signs. Usually fatal.	Antibiotics. Human hazard, so usually not treated.
Septicemia (many bacteria)	Blood poisoning. Fever, depression, shock. Often fatal.	Antibiotics. Treat shock. Supportive and symptomatic.
Histoplasmosis (fungus)	Diarrhea, coughing, eye discharge. All tissues may be affected. Respond if not too advanced.	Antibiotics. Supportive and symptomatic.

Other Infectious Diseases of Dogs (*continued*)

Cause	Symptoms/Prognosis	Treatment
Blastomycosis (fungus)	Coughing, skin and bone abscesses, eye discharge. All tissues may be affected. Respond if not too advanced.	As above.
Cryptococcosis (fungus)	Brain disease signs, skin and bone lesions, coughing. Respond if not too advanced.	As above.
Coccidioidomycosis (fungus)	Coughing, bone lesions. All tissues may be affected. Respond if not too advanced.	As above.
Nocardiosis and Actinomycosis (fungi)	Skin abscesses, coughing. Respond if not too advanced.	As above.

RESPIRATORY SYSTEM DISEASES

Unlike humans and cats, dogs seldom suffer from respiratory disease. The human cold syndrome of runny nose, scratchy eyes, sneezing, sore throat, etc. is not often seen in dogs. There are a number of infectious viral and bacterial respiratory diseases in dogs, but most are not serious unless there is an overwhelming infection from a combination of these organisms. Puppies, dogs in poor general condition, or those with other debilitating diseases are most susceptible to upper and lower respiratory system diseases.

Rhinitis

Rhinitis is an inflammation of the nasal passages, and can be acute or chronic. The causes most frequently encountered are: as an accompaniment to other diseases, such as distemper and pneumonia; bacterial, viral, and fungal respiratory infec-

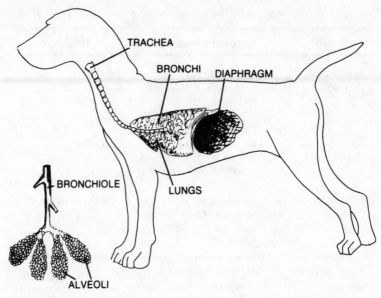

The Respiratory System

tions; trauma or injury; foreign bodies; tumors; allergies; congenital defects of the nose; poor nutrition; tooth and sinus infections; and nasal parasites.

SYMPTOMS   The symptoms of rhinitis are obvious to the dog owner, and include a watery or pustular nasal discharge, sneezing, open-mouth breathing, snorting, a moist cough, and sometimes fever.

DIAGNOSIS   The diagnosis is made by the symptoms, and a veterinary physical examination. It may be necessary to anesthetize the dog and examine the nasal cavities to determine the cause in some cases or to remove a foreign body. Culture and sensitivity testing of the discharges may be required in chronic cases to determine the antibiotic to use in treatment.

TREATMENT   Treatment is aimed at removing the primary cause. Antibiotics, corticosteroids, and nose drops may be used in infectious or allergic cases.

Sinusitis

Sinusitis is an infection or inflammation of the sinus cavities, most usually the frontal sinuses (above the eyes at the top of the nose) or the maxillary sinuses (below the eyes in the cheek area). Sinusitis is not a common problem in dogs. It is associated with extension of infection from the respiratory tract; tumors; infection of the roots of the upper fourth premolar tooth; and nasal foreign bodies and parasites.

SYMPTOMS The main sign of sinusitis in dogs is a nasal discharge, which may be just on one side of the nose. There is often an accompanying eye infection and discharge. Sometimes there is swelling over the affected sinus, and in cases caused by an infected tooth root penetrating the sinus, it is not unusual for the bone over the sinus to break down, resulting in a pus discharge flowing down the cheek.

DIAGNOSIS The diagnosis of sinusitis is made from the symptoms and physical examination; confirmation by x-rays may be necessary. Culture and sensitivity testing may need to be done on the discharges, particularly in chronic cases, to determine the antibiotic to use in treatment.

TREATMENT Treatment is aimed at removing the cause. Antibiotics, administered both orally and locally, are required in most cases. Surgical draining of the affected sinus may be recommended in chronic cases.

Tonsillitis

Tonsillitis is an inflammation of the tonsils, which are made up of lymphoid tissue and are thought to play an important role in preventing microorganisms from entering the body. Tonsillitis occurs quite frequently in dogs and the primary cause is a bacterial infection, usually a streptococcal organism. It also occurs secondarily to many other diseases, especially those of the respiratory tract. Tonsillar tumors are not uncommon in dogs. Some types of tonsillitis are contagious to other dogs.

SYMPTOMS Tonsillitis can be acute or chronic. The acute symptoms are loss of appetite, fever, difficulty swallowing, drooling, enlarged neck lymph nodes, and vomiting. Chronic cases have less severe symptoms.

DIAGNOSIS Diagnosis is made by the symptoms and if the dog cooperates, the veterinarian can look at the tonsil region to confirm the diagnosis. Some dogs will not allow their mouths to be opened, particularly if they are in pain, and they may have to be sedated for a thorough examination.

TREATMENT Treatment involves the use of antibiotics, a soft diet or subcutaneous or intravenous fluids if the dog is severely ill and not eating. Pain relievers may be required in some cases. Chronic cases may need to have the tonsils removed surgically.

Laryngitis

Laryngitis is an inflammation of the larynx and is seldom a serious problem in dogs. The most common cause in dogs is excessive barking. Other causes are respiratory infections, foreign bodies, or inhaled irritants.

SYMPTOMS The clinical signs of laryngitis in dogs are the same as those in people—loss of or change in the voice (hoarseness), coughing if pressure is applied to the larynx, difficulty in swallowing, and a bad odor to the breath.

DIAGNOSIS The diagnosis is made by the symptoms and a physical examination. Serious cases may require the use of an anesthetic to examine the throat.

TREATMENT Most cases get better without treatment, particularly if due to excessive barking. Antibiotics are used if the cause is a bacterial infection. Supportive care includes the use of soft food, warm quarters, pain relievers if needed, and steam inhalation.

Tracheitis and Bronchitis (Tracheobronchitis)

The trachea (windpipe) is the relatively rigid tube which extends from the larynx to the lungs. The bronchi are the large air passages of the lungs. Inflammation of the linings of the trachea and bronchi is referred to as tracheitis and bronchitis, respectively. As both are usually inflamed together, the condition is often referred to as tracheobronchitis. It can be acute or chronic.

Causes of acute tracheobronchitis are:

1. Viruses.
2. Bacteria.
3. Inhaled irritants.
4. Parasites.
5. Foreign bodies.
6. Trauma.

Causes of chronic tracheobronchitis are:

1. Acute cases that do not respond fully to treatment, or that receive no treatment.
2. Allergies.
3. As a secondary infection in other chronic respiratory or organ system diseases.

Infectious Tracheobronchitis (Kennel Cough): Tracheobronchitis caused by infectious viral or bacterial organisms can be a highly contagious disease of dogs and is particularly prevalent where dogs are housed together. It is often called kennel cough in such instances. Because it is seldom possible for a veterinary practitioner to identify the exact organism (and there is usually more than one) causing kennel cough, this is a general name for all infectious lower respiratory system diseases in dogs.

SYMPTOMS The symptoms include loss of appetite, depression, fever, vomiting in some cases, and a chronic, deep-chested cough. Kennel cough results in a distressing harsh, dry cough which can last more than a month, increasing in severity if the dog is exercised. Most dogs are not very ill with kennel cough, but severe infections with multiple organisms, particularly if not treated, can lead to pneumonia.

DIAGNOSIS Infectious tracheobronchitis usually includes a history of the affected dog mixing with other dogs. Diagnosis is made by the symptoms and a veterinary physical examination. In serious cases, x-rays and blood tests will be required to differentiate between bronchitis and pneumonia, as this can be difficult based on clinical signs alone. Culture and sensitivity testing may be recommended in cases which do not respond readily to treatment.

TREATMENT Dogs with infectious tracheobronchitis or kennel cough are highly contagious and should not be taken directly into the waiting room of a veterinary hospital. Check with the receptionist on how the hospital handles such cases, as most veterinary hospitals have isolation wards and examination rooms, removed from the general hospital area, for such contagious cases. Veterinary hospitals sometimes have to close down if an outbreak of kennel cough occurs, so all veterinarians take multiple precautions to avoid such outbreaks and appreciate cooperation in this endeavor.

Treatment is directed at preventing complications, as most cases resolve with supportive and symptomatic care. Antibiotics, cough suppressants, bronchodilators, and expectorants are used in treatment. Exercise should be restricted and the dog should be kept in warm, dry quarters. Serious cases will require hospitalization and the administration of fluids. Most dogs recover without complications if given supportive care, but the cough may persist for more than a month. Unless the cough worsens and the dog is depressed and not eating, owners should not worry about the slow recovery, as this is characteristic of kennel cough.

In noninfectious tracheobronchitis, treatment is directed at the cause such as: worming for parasites, endoscopic or surgical removal of a foreign body, and surgical repair, if necessary, of trauma. Chronic cases will require continuing treatment, and if allergic in origin, corticosteroids may be necessary.

PREVENTION Vaccines are now available for three of the

most common infectious agents involved in kennel cough: adenovirus type 2, *Bordetella,* and parainfluenza (*see also* Infectious Diseases for Which Vaccines Are Available, earlier in this chapter). Vaccinations help to prevent outbreaks of kennel cough, and are recommended for all dogs, but particularly for those that are going to be boarded or hospitalized.

Pneumonia

Pneumonia is an inflammation or infection of the lungs. The causes of pneumonia are numerous, including: bacterial and viral infectious agents that cause tracheobronchitis; fungal infections; foreign bodies; parasites; tumors; trauma; and as a secondary infection in many other diseases, such as heart failure.

SYMPTOMS The symptoms are similar to bronchitis, but much more severe. Shortness of breath and pain are also usually evident.

DIAGNOSIS Diagnosis is made by the symptoms, a physical examination, and lung sounds, and is confirmed by blood tests and x-rays. Culture and sensitivity testing is necessary in some cases.

TREATMENT Pneumonia, despite antibiotics, is often a fatal disease. All dogs with pneumonia require initial hospital treatment, which includes the use of oxygen and intravenous fluids in severe cases. Other treatments are similar to those used for severe bronchitis and will vary depending on the cause. If the pneumonia is secondary to other diseases or parasites, these will need to be treated also. Once the acute phase is over, continuing care can be given by the dog owner at home.

Dogs that have recovered from pneumonia may be more susceptible to respiratory infections and should be treated early if symptoms are evident. Some dogs may develop chronic bronchitis, which requires continuing care and treatment.

Other Respiratory Problems

The following respiratory problems occur in dogs. Most are complications from acute or chronic respiratory diseases, other organ system diseases or medical problems, or trauma.

- *Pulmonary edema* is an abnormal accumulation of fluid in the lungs. The most common cause in dogs is from left heart failure. Other causes are kidney failure, liver disease, tumors, poisons, severe allergic reaction, trauma, shock, and inhalation of irritants. Severe pulmonary edema is an emergency situation and requires immediate veterinary treatment with oxygen, bronchodilators, diuretics, pain relievers, and corticosteroids. The primary disease or injury causing the pulmonary edema will also need to be treated.
- *Bronchiectasis* is an abnormal dilation of the bronchial tubes; it occurs secondarily to other respiratory diseases.
- *Emphysema* is an overinflation of the air sacs or the tissues between them, which prevents air from readily escaping from the lungs. It occurs in chronic respiratory diseases.
- *Atelectasis* is an incomplete expansion or collapse of the lungs. It occurs in chronic respiratory diseases.
- *Pleurisy* is an inflammation of the membranes lining the outside of the lungs and the inside of the chest wall. It usually accompanies other acute respiratory diseases, such as pneumonia.
- *Pyothorax* is the presence of pus in the pleural cavity, which is the space between the outer lining of the lungs and the inner lining of the chest wall. The causes are the spread of infection from the lungs or through the blood from other areas of the body, or from penetrating wounds of the chest.
- *Hemothorax* is the presence of blood in the pleural cavity. The most common cause is trauma.

- *Pneumothorax* is the presence of air in the pleural cavity. The cause is usually traumatic, resulting from penetrating wounds of the chest or rupture of the lungs or airways.

ENDOCRINE (HORMONAL) SYSTEM DISEASES AND DISORDERS

The endocrine system is made up of endocrine glands, which secrete substances called hormones into the blood that influence metabolism and other body processes. Metabolism is the sum total of all the physical and chemical activities by which life processes are maintained. The major malfunctions of these glands that affect the dog have been discussed in other sections. The endocrine glands, their location, normal functions, and abnormal functions (*hyper* is excessive and *hypo* is deficient) are:

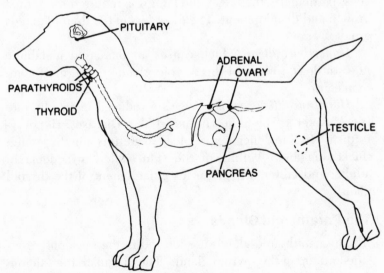

The Endocrine (Hormonal) Glands

The Pituitary Gland

The pituitary gland is located at the base of the brain. This gland produces a number of different hormones, affecting the function of all the other glands. Excessive production of one hormone, called the growth hormone, leads to giant size; deficiency leads to dwarf size. The major signs of malfunction of the pituitary relate to the effects on the other glands. Hypofunction can lead to a disease called *diabetes insipidus,* which results in the production of excessive quantities of dilute urine; however, this disease should not be confused with *diabetes mellitus,* which is caused by insufficiency of a hormone called insulin produced by the pancreas.

The Thyroid Glands

The thyroid glands are located in the neck on either side of the trachea (windpipe). These glands require sufficient quantities of iodine for normal production of the thyroid hormone. The thyroid hormone affects the metabolism of all tissues, particularly the metabolic rate; it is required for normal growth and development. The disorders of the thyroid glands are:

Hyperthyroidism, which causes an increased metabolic rate. In dogs, tumors of the thyroid gland are the most common cause.

Hypothyroidism, which causes a reduced metabolic rate (*see* Chapter 4, The Skin; Hormonal Skin Diseases: Hypothyroidism). Iodine deficiency can lead to cretinism in the young; thickening and swelling of the skin, called myxedema in adults; and goiter, which causes enlargement of the thyroid glands.

The Parathyroid Glands

The parathyroid glands are located in the neck on the inside and top of the thyroid glands. They regulate the calcium in the blood and tissues. Disorders of this pair of glands are:

Hyperparathyroidism, which causes an increased blood calcium and can be caused by tumors or disease of the glands, but is more commonly due to kidney disease or diet imbalances in dogs (*see* Chapter 1, Nutrition; All-Meat Diet).

Hypoparathyroidism, which causes a deficiency of blood calcium (*see* Chapter 16, Emergency Care; Emergency Cases: Eclampsia).

The Adrenal Glands

The adrenal glands are located in the abdomen above the kidneys. These glands control carbohydrate, fat, and protein metabolism; water and salt balances; and sex hormones. Disorders are:

Hyperadrenocorticism. Also called Cushing's syndrome (*see* Chapter 4, The Skin; Hormonal Skin Diseases: Hyperadrenocorticism; *also* Chapter 17, Drugs; Veterinary Drugs: Corticosteroids).

Hypoadrenocorticism. Also called Addison's disease (*see* Chapter 17, Drugs; Veterinary Drugs: Corticosteroids).

The Gonads or Sex Glands

The gonads or sex glands (testicles in the male and ovaries in the female) are located in the abdomen. Disorders are:

Hyperfunction. Male (rare). Female (*see* Chapter 4, The Skin; Hormonal Skin Diseases: Female Dogs—Sex Hormone Problems, Hyperestrogenism).

Hypofunction. Male (*see* Chapter 4, The Skin; Hormonal Skin Diseases: Male Dogs—Sex Hormone Problems). Female (*see* Chapter 4, The Skin; Hormonal Skin Diseases: Female Dogs—Sex Hormone Problems, Hypoestrogenism).

The Pancreas

The pancreas is located in the abdomen, behind the stomach. This gland produces insulin, which regulates the body's use and blood level of sugar. Disorders are:

Hyperfunction. Seldom a problem in dogs, but seen in some tumors of the pancreas. It leads to hypoglycemia.

Hypofunction. Diabetes mellitus (*see* following description).

Diabetes Mellitus

In diabetes mellitus body chemistry is affected because certain cells of the pancreas no longer secrete the insulin needed to regulate the body's use of carbohydrates. This results in high blood sugar and sugar in the urine. The cause may be identified as a disease or tumor of the pancreas, but in most cases the cause is unknown. There are a number of predisposing factors, including heredity, obesity, and the use of corticosteroids.

SYMPTOMS   The disease is relatively common in dogs and is seen most frequently in older female dogs of the smaller breeds.

Early signs are:

• Increased urination.
• Increased water intake.
• Increased appetite.
• Weight loss.
• Increased susceptibility to infections.
• Poor wound healing.

Later signs are:

• Vomiting.
• Diarrhea.
• Weakness.
• Cataracts.
• Coma.

DIAGNOSIS   The diagnosis is made by the history and clinical signs and is confirmed by laboratory tests, which show sugar in the urine and high blood sugar levels. Other diagnostic tests may also be required.

TREATMENT There is no cure, but diabetes can be controlled with treatment. Treatment involves injections of insulin daily, regulation of the amount and type of food, and a controlled amount of exercise. In dogs the disease is usually well advanced when diagnosed, so the diet regulation and oral drugs useful in humans are seldom effective in treatment.

Hospital treatment. Initially, a veterinarian will need to treat a diabetic dog to bring its body chemistry back to normal and to determine the type of diet and amount of insulin needed for maintenance.

The dog will also need to be checked by a veterinarian at regular intervals to make sure the diabetes is being satisfactorily controlled.

Home care. Following a diagnosis of diabetes in a dog and the initial veterinary treatment, a dog owner can then care for the dog at home, treating the disease as follows:

Insulin. The veterinarian will show the dog owner how to give the daily insulin injections relatively painlessly with special insulin syringes and needles. Morning administration is usually recommended, as it takes several hours before the peak activity of the insulin occurs. Some dogs with severe diabetes may require more than one injection daily.

Diet. A balanced, readily available, good-grade dog food will be recommended to ensure that the same levels of fats, carbohydrates, and proteins are consumed daily. The nutritional requirements of a diabetic dog are the same as those of a normal dog, but a uniform diet is most important in controlling diabetes in the dog once an insulin dosage has been established. A low carbohydrate diet is no longer recommended in controlling diabetes, but a constant carbohydrate input each day is necessary, so the dog's food must not be changed. The food should be fed throughout the day to reduce the possibility of overloading the ability of the body to control the blood glucose level. A suggested feeding regimen is one quarter of the daily food in the morning, one half at midday, and the remaining one quarter in the evening.

Daily routine. Exercise, environmental temperatures, stress, etc., all affect the amount of insulin required daily, so dogs with diabetes should lead very regular, routine lives. Females should be spayed, as estrus and pregnancy are stressful and affect the insulin requirements.

Urine testing. The dog owner will need to regularly test the urine with a test tape which will be dispensed by the veterinarian, to determine if sugar is being passed in the urine. If sugar is present in more than small amounts, adjustments will need to be made in the insulin dosage, but the dog owner should check with the veterinarian before making any dosage changes.

Monitoring. The diabetic dog must be watched closely for signs of lack of blood sugar regulation. If insufficient insulin is given, the early signs of the disease will recur. On the other hand, increased hunger, nervousness, weakness, and convulsions indicate that too much insulin is being given, causing low blood sugar. The dog owner will need to give the dog some sugar immediately to avoid a serious insulin shock reaction.

Most owners of diabetic dogs become very informed about the disease. Once they get over the initial shock of having to give injections, they do not find it too much trouble. The cost of maintenance is not high, and periodic check-ups of the dog by a veterinarian should be nominal.

15
Cancer

Medical Terms Used to Describe Cancer

The words "cancer," "tumor," and "neoplasm" are used interchangeably in discussions of cancer, and this has become an acceptable practice. By definition, however, their meanings are:

Tumor. A tumor is a swelling; today it is a commonly used word for a cancerous growth. Not all cancers are tumors, however; leukemia, for example, is a cancer of the blood. Tumors can be benign or malignant.

Neoplasm. A neoplasm is a new and abnormal growth.

Cancer. Cancer is a malignant tumor or neoplasm. Cancer transforms a living cell into a cancer cell, which then takes over control of the cell's growth and functions. Cancer cells invade and destroy normal tissue, spread to other areas of the body, multiply much more frequently than normal cells, and transmit all these abnormalities to succeeding generations of cancer cells. The natural course of cancer, without treatment, is fatal.

Benign or Malignant

A tumor can be benign or malignant. The following chart outlines the characteristics of both types of tumors, although the division is by no means clear-cut. A tumor can be benign,

Tumors

Benign	Malignant
• Rounded and encapsulated	• Irregular growth
• Lymph nodes not involved	• Lymph nodes involved
• In one location	• Multiple locations
• Slow or no growth	• Rapid growth
• Does not spread	• Metastasis—spread or seed to other body locations
Cause damage by occupying space, which can interfere with function of other nearby body tissues	Cause damage by occupying space and invading and destroying normal tissues

malignant, both benign and malignant, and occasionally a benign tumor can become malignant.

Cancer is a relatively common disease in dogs over five years of age, and the incidence increases with advancing age. There is a higher incidence of tumors in dogs than in cats, but in cats about 80% are malignant, whereas in dogs only about 35% are malignant. This is because the most common site for dog tumors (about 40%) is the skin, and in cats it is the highly malignant leukemia complex cancers that are most common. The next most common site for tumors in dogs are the mammary glands, and about 50% of these are malignant, although they seldom occur in spayed females or male dogs, and these are followed in incidence by tumors of the digestive tract and by lymphosarcomas. Purebred dogs have a higher incidence of cancer than dogs of mixed breeds.

Symptoms and Diagnosis of Cancer

Early diagnosis of cancer is difficult in dogs, but should be suspected in any older dog that suffers gradual loss of weight, loss of appetite, and weakness. Dog owners should watch for signs of cancer as outlined in the following chart:

DIAGNOSIS   If a dog shows any slow loss in condition, or

Symptoms of Cancer in Dogs

Location	Symptoms
Skin	Tumor or lump evident. An ulcerated or bleeding wound which does not heal. Not usually painful.
Mammary gland	Small, hard lump under skin, at or near teat. May ulcerate and bleed.
Digestive system	Loss of weight and appetite. Vomiting. Constipation or diarrhea with blood.
Urinary system	Blood in urine. Excessive or painful urination. No urination.
Genital system	Male (Prostate): Stiff gait. Difficult urination or defecation. Pain. Female: Uterine bleeding. Enlarged abdomen. Digestive upsets.
Blood system	Enlarged lymph nodes. Loss of weight and appetite. Anemia.
Bone	Swelling, lameness, and pain.
Nose	Bloody or chronic mucous discharge. Sneezing. Pain.
Mouth	Reluctance to eat. Growths or sores in mouth. Salivation. Pain.
Eye	Swelling. Pain. Loss of vision.
Lung	Coughing and shortness of breath.
Liver	Loss of weight and appetite. Vomiting. Abdominal swelling from fluid. Tender abdomen. Jaundice (yellowing).
Pancreas	Loss of weight and appetite. Digestive upsets. Jaundice. Abdominal pain.
Nervous system	Incoordination. Seizures. Head pressing. Disturbance of vision. Paralysis.
Glands (Hormone)	Pituitary and adrenals: Excessive thirst and urination. Loss of hair and darkening of skin. Enlarged abdomen. Thyroid: Lump in neck. May be painful. Ovaries: Upset in estrus cycle. If large, then difficult urination and digestive upsets. Testes: Enlargement of testicle. Pain. Feminization signs.
Heart	Symptoms of heart failure.

any of the warning signs listed in the accompanying chart, it should be taken to a veterinarian for a check-up. A diagnosis of cancer requires some or all of the following:

- A complete medical history with emphasis on recent signs.
- A physical examination.
- Blood tests.
- X-rays to locate an internal tumor or check if the cancer has spread.
- In some cases, exploratory surgery will be required to make a diagnosis.
- The diagnosis of cancer will need to be confirmed by having discharges and/or biopsy tissues examined microscopically by a veterinary pathologist.

When a complete diagnosis has been made, your veterinarian can advise you on the prognosis, and whether or not treatment is practical or possible.

Treatment of Cancer

Diagnosis of cancer tends to be made later in dogs than in humans, which makes it more difficult to treat. However, the choice does not always have to be euthanasia. Many dog cancers respond very well to surgical and/or medical treatments. A one-year survival in a dog is equivalent to five years in a human, if you take the differing average life spans into account. With treatment, prolongation of life is possible in most cases, with cure in some cases; and spontaneous complete regression does occur occasionally.

Before recommending treatment your veterinarian will need to determine the dog's general medical condition; the specific cancer and whether it is localized or has spread; the treatments available and their effectiveness for this type of cancer; the dog owner's wishes concerning treatment; the time and extent of treatment needed; the cost; the quality of life for the dog during and after treatment; and the prognosis.

Treatments for cancer in dogs are the same as those used

in people, and include: surgery, radiation, chemotherapy, immunotherapy, hormones, supportive and symptomatic treatment, and combinations of some or all of these.

Laetrile and Cancer

Many dog owners ask veterinarians if laetrile is a useful cancer treatment. Laetrile, which is a compound extracted from apricot pits, is poisonous in high dosages; a number of human deaths have been attributed to its use. Several extensive studies have found that the toxic agent, a cyanide, approached poisonous levels, which were considered unsafe when used as its advocates advise.

Many people with cancer who claim to have been helped or cured by laetrile treatment have had prior radiation treatment or chemotherapy, and the response noted while on laetrile is the delayed response to these therapies. It must also be remembered that not all cancers advance. Some are destroyed or suppressed by the body's immune system, and a natural cure or remission occurs. It is now theorized that people and animals are subject to attack by cancers every day, but that individuals with healthy immune systems destroy these abnormal cancer cells, and it is only those with depressed immune systems who succumb to the disease. According to all the most reliable authorities, laetrile is not effective in the treatment of cancer. The National Cancer Institute, the Mayo Clinic, the University of California at Los Angeles, Memorial Sloan-Kettering, and the University of Arizona have done extensive studies, all of which found that laetrile appeared to have no antitumor effects on several types of cancer, even when combined with the vitamins and special diets recommended by its proponents.

16
Emergency Care

EMERGENCY CASES

It is important for a dog owner to be able to recognize when an ill or injured dog needs emergency treatment.

SIGNS AND SYMPTOMS Any of the following signs and symptoms constitutes an emergency, and the dog needs immediate veterinary treatment:

- Unconsciousness.
- Shock.
- Hemorrhaging (bleeding) profusely.
- Severe respiratory distress.
- Cardiac arrest.
- Convulsions (seizures) that are continuous or last more than five minutes.
- High fever—over 106° Fahrenheit.
- Severe depression.
- Severe vomiting.
- No urination, particularly if attempts are made to urinate.

TREATMENT In emergencies a dog owner can attempt to stop external bleeding with the use of pressure bandages or cloths, or use a tourniquet if a limb or the tail is involved. The owner can also administer cardiopulmonary resuscitation if required. However, the most essential thing is to get the dog to a veterinary hospital as quickly as possible. Immediate lifesaving veterinary treatment is most important in emergencies, and delay lessens the chances of saving the dog. Emergency measures will include some or all of the following:

1. Clear the airway if obstructed and insert a tube into the trachea (windpipe), or, if necessary, perform a tracheotomy (incision made in the trachea through the skin and muscles of the neck). If the dog is not breathing, mechanical respiration equipment should be connected.

2. Treat cardiac arrest using cardiopulmonary resuscitation measures, drugs, and defibrillation (electroshock) if necessary.

3. Stop hemorrhaging by pressure, tourniquet, or surgery if required.

4. Administer oxygen.

5. Administer intravenous blood, plasma, or fluids.

6. Treat shock.

7. Immobilize fractures temporarily.

8. Relieve pain.

Once the dog's condition is stabilized, history taking, diagnostic tests, and evaluation of injuries or diseases can be done. Treatment and prognosis can then be discussed with the dog owner.

Shock

As used medically, the word "shock" is not well understood by the public. People frequently use this word to describe their reaction to bad news or to a catastrophe of some sort. This type of emotional reaction has nothing to do with the medical meaning of shock, which is a serious and life-threatening medical condition.

Shock is a medical term used to describe a state of blood distribution collapse, which results in failure of the blood flow to body tissues and vital organs, thereby depriving them of oxygen and the removal of wastes. Often, despite medical care and the apparent absence of serious injury, shock can result in death. The exact cause is unknown, but shock occurs when the body is exposed to serious medical problems, such as accidents; heart failure; hemorrhage; burns; advanced infections; dehydration; acute allergic reactions; advanced cancers; and poisonings.

SYMPTOMS In shock the body attempts to compensate for the poor blood circulation by increasing the heart rate and constricting the blood vessels of the extremities. Thus, the symptoms of shock are:

- Collapse.
- Rapid and weak or absent pulse.
- Rapid heart and respiratory rate.
- Pallor (in dogs this can be seen in the gum color).
- Low body temperature, especially of the extremities (the legs and paws feel cold).
- Thirst if conscious.
- Low blood pressure.

If the body cannot compensate sufficiently or treatment cannot overcome the symptoms, the shock becomes irreversible and death soon follows.

DIAGNOSIS Diagnosis is made by the history, symptoms, and a veterinary physical examination, and is confirmed by laboratory tests.

TREATMENT An animal in shock needs immediate veterinary medical care. In an emergency, the dog owner can take the following first aid measures:

1. Place the dog on its side on a blanket.
2. Raise the hindquarters with a pillow to increase blood flow to the heart.
3. Pull out the tongue to ensure the airway is not obstructed.
4. Stop any hemorrhage, if possible, with pressure, using a gauze pad or clean cloth; do not use a tourniquet unless blood is spurting from a limb or the tail, and if used do not apply too tightly or for more than fifteen minutes.
5. Use a hot water bottle or blanket to keep the dog warm.
6. Transport to a veterinary hospital as soon as possible.

Hospital treatment is aimed at restoring the blood volume with transfusions of blood, plasma, and/or electrolytes. Corticosteroids, antibiotics, pain killers, drugs which act on the blood vessels, and other supportive measures are needed on an emergency basis to save an animal in shock.

Cardiopulmonary Resuscitation

Cardiac emergencies occur when the heart stops beating or beats inadequately. Pulmonary emergencies occur when breathing stops or is seriously depressed. Only one of these may occur, but usually both occur together and a cardiopulmonary emergency then exists. If resuscitation or revival measures are not taken within five minutes, the dog will be dead.

Cardiopulmonary resuscitation (CPR) is a technique both of external cardiac massage, which keeps the blood circulating, and of artificial respiration, which delivers oxygen to the lungs.

Cardiopulmonary resuscitation is similar in humans and dogs, although there are minor differences in technique and timing.

The unconscious dog should be laid on its right side. If a heartbeat cannot be detected or there is no respiration, then begin CPR.

Pulmonary Resuscitation. Make sure the airway is not obstructed. Hold the dog's mouth and lips closed and lift the head. The person applying the CPR should then take a deep breath, place his or her mouth over the dog's nose, and blow until the dog's chest rises, or resistance is felt. The person should then remove his or her mouth and allow the chest to fall of its own accord. This should be repeated eight to twelve times every sixty seconds. It may require two or three breaths each time to inflate the chest of a large dog.

Cardiac Resuscitation. The dog's heart is located about two inches behind the elbow when leg is extended (varies with dog). (A dog owner should become familiar with the location under normal conditions because it cannot, of course,

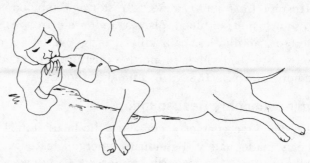

Technique for Pulmonary Resuscitation

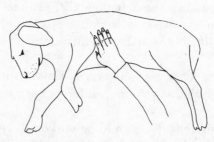

Technique for Cardiac or Heart Resuscitation

be located if there is no heartbeat.) With the dog lying on its right side, on a firm surface, a person should place the palm of his or her hand over the heart, press firmly, then release. (Both hands may be needed to get enough compression in a large dog.) This should be done once every second, or sixty times a minute. The compression should be held for a count of two and released for a count of one.

When giving CPR to a dog, one breath is required for every five heart compressions. If possible, two people should apply CPR, one for the cardiac massage and the other to give artificial respiration.

If the dog is small, there is less likely to be damage to the chest if the rescuer grasps the chest so that the palm of the hand is under the chest below the heart, and the thumb is over the chest above the heart. Compression can then be applied by squeezing the thumb and fingers together.

One should check frequently to see if the dog is breathing or has a heartbeat. The femoral pulse can be felt on the inside of the back leg about midway between the knee and the hip joint. Meanwhile, still maintaining CPR, get the dog to a veterinarian. If veterinary care is unavailable and the dog does not respond after thirty minutes, further efforts are seldom worthwhile.

Heat Stroke

Heat stroke is a disturbance of the heat-regulating mechanism of the body. The most common causes of heat stroke in dogs are a high environmental temperature, high humidity, and poor ventilation. Heat stroke is common not only in very hot weather but also on 75° days if a dog is left in an unventilated closed area, such as a car. It may even happen when a dog is suddenly transported from a temperate to a hot climate.

In dogs, it is not so much the air temperature as lack of air circulation that causes heat stroke. Static air near a dog's body quickly rises to the dog's body temperature; this blocks further heat dissipation. Therefore, a continuous change of air enveloping the dog's body—that is, good ventilation—is important in hot weather.

Dogs do not sweat through their skin as people do. Body temperature reduction and temperature control in dogs are achieved by vaporizing large volumes of water from their lungs. This is speeded up by panting, which increases the respiratory rate and reduces the depth of each breath.

The body temperature in heat stroke can quickly rise as high as 109° Fahrenheit (normal in the dog is 101.5°). If a dog is subjected to heat for too long and the body temperature rises, it will lose consciousness, and can quickly die.

Dog owners need to pay close attention to puppies, short-nosed dogs, fat dogs, and older dogs in hot weather because they are particularly susceptible to heat stroke.

SYMPTOMS The symptoms of heat stroke include:

- Loud panting.
- Difficulty in breathing.
- Increased heart rate.
- Vomiting.
- Red gums.
- A frightened or staring expression.

TREATMENT The immediate emergency treatment for heat stroke is to get the dog out of the heat and then place it in a bath of cold water to get the temperature down—*fast*. If a bath is not available, use a spray from a hose, pour water from a container, or sponge the dog down repeatedly. Once a dog has been brought out of the acute stage of heat stroke, veterinary examination and treatment are recommended as relapses are not uncommon.

PREVENTION Common sense prevents heat stroke in dogs. Remember—whenever a person feels hot, a dog feels equally hot. The following precautions are recommended during hot weather conditions:

1. Do not exercise a dog strenuously on a hot day.
2. Dogs will seek shade on a hot day, so make sure shade is available. Remember that the sun's position changes rapidly in summer, so be sure the dog can continually move into shade.
3. Provide plenty of cold water, whether at home or traveling.
4. If it is unbearably hot, place a wet towel on the dog.
5. Feed early in the morning or late in the evening.
6. Lastly, but most important, NEVER leave a dog in a closed car, or even in a ventilated car, for more than a few minutes in the heat. If the dog must be left in the car, try to park in the shade and leave all the windows open.

Electrocution

Electrocution is the passage of an electric current through the body. The most common cause of electrocution in dogs is from chewing on electric cords. Considering that nearly all puppies chew on electrical cords, serious injury is surprisingly rare. One very rare cause of electrocution in dogs is from being hit by lightning, and in most of these instances, death is instantaneous.

SYMPTOMS   The usual injury from such encounters is a slight electric shock or an electrical burn on the tongue, mouth, or lips. These burns have a grayish appearance and most heal without complications, although the dog may be reluctant to eat for a day or two.

If a severe electric shock is received, the dog will collapse and stiffen immediately. Once the cord is unplugged and removed from the mouth, the dog will regain consciousness in most cases, but some seizure activity may occur during the recovery stage.

TREATMENT   The first thing a dog owner should do if such an electrical accident occurs is to unplug the cord before removing it from the dog's mouth. If the cord is removed without unplugging it, the dog owner may also be electrocuted.

If the dog has no heartbeat or is not breathing, cardiopulmonary resuscitation should be started. The recovered dog should be checked for mouth burns and watched closely for the next several days. If the dog does not recover quickly, or if any signs of breathing difficulty occur after recovery, veterinary treatment should be sought at once.

PROGNOSIS   Most dogs survive if the owner is present and quickly unplugs the cord. If no one is present, respiratory and heart failure will be fatal in a short time if the cord remains stuck to the dog's mouth.

Fortunately, most dogs stop chewing things when they mature. Many young dogs receive minor electrical shocks from such activity and quickly learn to leave electric cords alone. Strict discipline for such activity will help prevent electrical injuries.

Frostbite

Frostbite is damage to the tissues from exposure to low temperatures. Frostbite is not an uncommon injury in dogs left outside in cold climates.

SYMPTOMS   In frostbite, the extremities are most often involved—the ears, tail tip, and feet. The affected areas are firm, pale, and bloodless; on rewarming they become red, swollen, and painful.

TREATMENT   Treatment today is by quickly rewarming the affected areas in a water bath or pack at 105° to 108° Fahrenheit (not above 110°) for fifteen to twenty minutes; the old methods of slow rewarming and rubbing with snow are no longer recommended. Warm drinks, hot water bottles, and heating pads are also helpful.

After rewarming and cleaning the affected areas, an antiseptic dressing or ointment should be applied. Gentle daily massage helps circulation. In most cases the skin will peel rather like a sunburn and then heal. In severe frostbite the skin may turn dark, shrivel, and fall away, but if infection occurs or the area involved is large, surgical removal may be required.

PREVENTION   Dogs left outside in the winter should have shelter, and if the temperatures are well below freezing, heated quarters are recommended. The windchill factor must also be taken into account. Extra food is needed to maintain body temperature in the cold—up to three times as much as normal. Fatigue, young or old age, illness, and altitude also affect susceptibility to frostbite. Outdoor dogs should be checked daily in cold weather by examining their ears and tails for signs of frostbite.

Acute Peritonitis

Peritonitis is an inflammation of the peritoneum which is the inside lining of the abdominal cavity wall and the outside lining of the organs contained within the abdominal cavity. Fluids, organic debris, cells, infectious organisms, and pus accumulate in the cavity in acute peritonitis. Without treatment, it can be fatal quickly. The causes can be from external injury or internal infections or diseases, such as bowel puncture from trauma or rupture from disease or ingested foreign bodies, with escape of contaminated bowel contents into the abdominal cavity; infections from abdominal cavity puncture, or postsurgically, or spreading from infections in other abdominal organs or other areas of the body; damage to the urinary system, with escape of urine into the abdominal cavity; damage to the pancreas or liver with escape of bile or pancreatic enzymes into the abdominal cavity; and rupture of an infected uterus or prostate gland.

SYMPTOMS Acute peritonitis is accompanied by severe pain and abdominal tenderness. The dog usually walks with a stiff gait and the abdominal muscles are rigid in an attempt to guard the abdomen. There is loss of appetite, vomiting, fever, increased heart and respiratory rate, and symptoms of shock develop in a few hours.

DIAGNOSIS The diagnosis is made by the symptoms, a physical examination, absence of bowel sounds, and evidence of fluid in the abdomen. X-rays and laboratory tests confirm the diagnosis. An abdominal fluid sample may be withdrawn and examined microscopically to assist in identifying the cause of the peritonitis. If bacterial infection is present, a culture and sensitivity test on the abdominal fluid to determine the antibiotic to use in treatment may be necessary.

TREATMENT Treatment is directed at removing the cause, and if organ rupture or perforation has occurred, surgery is essential to repair the injury or to drain an abscess. Antibiotics will be given to control infection. Treatment for shock and symptomatic and supportive care, including the use of pain relievers and intravenous feeding, will be required in most cases.

PROGNOSIS The prognosis depends on the severity of the peritonitis and on how quickly treatment is started.

Eclampsia (Puerperal Tetany, or Milk Fever)

Eclampsia is a condition that leads to convulsions and coma; it occurs most commonly in female dogs of the small breeds that are nursing a large litter. It usually occurs in the first two weeks after giving birth, but may occur before delivery or even in the weaning period. It is also called puerperal tetany; puerperal is the period after giving birth and tetany is a condition in which there is muscle twitching, cramps, and convulsions. Another older name is milk fever, as the condition was known to be related to lactation.

Eclampsia is caused by hypocalcemia, which is a low blood calcium level. Why this occurs in some dogs is unknown, but the demand for calcium during pregnancy and lactation can exhaust the calcium stores in the body and this may lead to hypocalcemia.

SYMPTOMS   The signs, in the order of progression, are:

- Restlessness.
- Panting.
- Anxiety.
- Whining.
- Drooling.
- Stiffness.
- Staggering.
- Twitching of muscles.
- Dilated pupils.
- Fever.
- Collapse.
- Convulsions or seizures.
- Death if not treated.

DIAGNOSIS   The diagnosis is readily made from the history of pregnancy or nursing and the symptoms. The blood calcium level can be determined by testing, but is only used to later confirm the diagnosis, as immediate treatment is essential.

TREATMENT Eclampsia responds dramatically to intravenous calcium injections. Unfortunately, relapses often occur, so an additional intramuscular injection of calcium is usually given, and if possible, the litter is taken away from the mother. The veterinarian will also advise on the diet for the mother and if additional calcium and vitamin D supplements are required.

PREVENTION Dogs that get eclampsia with one litter often get it again with later litters. To prevent recurrences, a good diet, which has adequate vitamin D and balanced amounts of calcium and phosphorus, is recommended during pregnancy and lactation. Corticosteroids appear to prevent recurrences in cases which do not respond to dietary control. Additional calcium during pregnancy and lactation may aggravate rather than prevent recurrences, so oversupplementation should be avoided.

Wounds

A wound is a cut or break in the skin. Most wounds in dogs are minor and do not constitute an emergency, but if the wound is large, bleeding, or accompanied by more serious injuries, immediate veterinary care is essential. The most common causes of wounds in dogs are from automobile accidents, bites from dog fights, and contact with broken glass or other sharp objects such as barbed wire.

SYMPTOMS Wounds cause pain and may result in hemorrhaging. Loss of function and infection may also occur. Dog owners can usually determine the severity of a wound by observation, and only those which are extensive, uncontrollably bleeding, or accompanied by signs of shock or other serious injury need immediate treatment.

TREATMENT Minor wounds can be treated by the dog owner. The wound should be cleaned with water, and then an antiseptic should be applied. Bandaging is seldom necessary or desirable unless the wound is in an area that is continually being further contaminated. Most minor wounds heal quickly in the dog, but the owner should inspect the wound daily to make sure that it is not becoming infected.

Major wounds will require surgical treatment to clean and close the wound, and to stop hemorrhaging. Antibiotics will be used to control infection. Pain relievers and treatment for shock may be required if the wounds are extensive or if there was severe blood loss or other complicating injuries. Large wounds in which there is extensive skin loss may require reconstruction or skin grafting.

Burns

A burn is destruction of the skin or deeper tissues caused by contact with heat or fire. Burns can be of different types and have the following causes: direct heat, such as scalding by hot liquids or grease, or burns from hot objects such as tar and heating pads; radiant heat, such as sun and heat lamps; flames, from fires; friction, from ropes or pavement; electricity, from electric wires or lightning; corrosive chemicals, such as acids, alkalis, and phenols; and smoke from fire.

SYMPTOMS Burns are usually broken down into the following categories:

First degree, or superficial, burns. These burns only involve the outer (epithelial) layer of the skin, which will be red, hot, and painful.

Second degree, or partial thickness, burns. These burns injure the skin and some of the deeper tissues. In addition to the signs of first degree burns, blisters or vesicles form, and there is swelling of the skin with later crusting of the involved areas.

Third degree, or full thickness, burns. These burns entirely destroy the superficial and deeper layers of the skin, which looks charred; later the destroyed skin ulcerates and sloughs (falls away), exposing the underlying tissues. While these burns are not as painful as the others, if extensive they can quickly lead to shock.

Smoke inhalation injury leads to signs of respiratory problems such as coughing and shortness of breath.

TREATMENT   Treatment depends on the cause, size, depth, and location of the burns, and on the age and general condition of the dog.

Unless extensive, first and second degree burns can usually be treated by the dog owner, initially by applying cold packs and then by keeping the area clean until healing occurs. It is usually best not to apply ointments or bandages in dogs as this only leads the dog to lick or tear at the lesions. If the dog will not let the burned area heal or infection occurs, veterinary treatment should be sought.

More extensive, or third degree, burns will require veterinary care. Antibiotics, pain relievers, fluids, and other supportive and symptomatic care will be required. In severe burn cases, treatment of shock and prevention of infection will be essential as these are the most dangerous complications in burn cases.

Full thickness burns will require surgical treatment which will entail removal of the burned skin in small lesions or the use of skin grafts in more extensive lesions. Hydrotherapy baths daily are helpful in removing the dead skin less painfully. Restraints and/or sedation are necessary in treating burns in dogs to prevent them from further mutilating the areas involved or interfering with skin grafts. Because treatment is prolonged, difficult, and expensive, most dogs with extensive burns over the body are euthanized.

Smoke inhalation treatment is directed at preventing the development of pneumonia.

PROGNOSIS   The prognosis depends on how much of the body surface is burned and on the thickness of the burn. A rough guide to prognosis is the percentage of body surface burned: If less than 15%, the chances are good; if 15% to 50%, they are fair; and greater than 50%, the survival rate is poor.

Radiation Injury

Radiation injury disrupts biological molecules which leads to death of cells. It is caused by ionizing radiation and can be the result of electromagnetic gamma or x-rays, which have no mass or charge and travel at the speed of light, or of particulate alpha or beta particles, which have mass and variable velocities.

SYMPTOMS The injury from radiation depends on the dose, amount absorbed, area exposed, and organs affected. Massive exposure, such as that from an atomic explosion, leads to instant death from the blast, or death in a few days or weeks from the effects of the radiation.

The rapidly dividing cells of the body are most sensitive to radiation and signs of injury become apparent when these destroyed cells are inadequately replaced. The first signs are evident in the blood tissues, followed by the intestines, and then the skin. Nerve and muscle cells do not divide in adults, so are not as affected by radiation.

Symptoms usually show up in a few days to a few weeks as the damage to the blood and immune systems becomes evident. Hemorrhaging, particularly noticeable in the skin, vomiting, bloody diarrhea, and overwhelming infections lead to death in about two weeks in heavy exposures. The severity of the symptoms depends on the exposure, and milder cases usually fully recover in three to four months.

Excessive non-lethal radiation can lead to developmental defects in the fetus or cause cancers, particularly leukemias.

DIAGNOSIS Diagnosis is made from the history of exposure to radiation, the symptoms, and a physical examination; it is confirmed by blood tests.

TREATMENT Treatment is supportive and symptomatic until the body can repair itself. Blood transfusions and bone marrow implants have been used in human cases of radiation injury with success. Antibiotics are used to control infections and fluids combat the dehydration that accompanies the vomiting and diarrhea.

Thoracic Trauma Emergencies

Thoracic trauma occurs when there is any injury to the chest cavity. The main emergencies which arise are pneumothorax, hemothorax, and diaphragmatic hernia. The most common causes of thoracic trauma emergencies in dogs are automobile accidents, dog fights, and falls from a height. Any of these injuries can lead to *pneumothorax*, which is the presence of air in the pleural cavity (the space between the outer lining of the lungs and the inner lining of the chest wall), either from a wound to the outside or from rupture of the airways or lungs; *hemothorax*, which is the presence of blood in the pleural cavity; or *diaphragmatic hernia*, which is a tear in the muscular partition separating the thoracic and abdominal cavities.

SYMPTOMS   If air or blood accumulates in the pleural cavity, it compresses the lungs and symptoms of difficulty in breathing or shortness of breath are evident. These are emergency situations and require immediate treatment. Diaphragmatic hernia is not always an emergency situation, but can be if the abdominal organs enter the thoracic cavity and compress the lungs and the heart.

DIAGNOSIS   The diagnosis is made from the history of an accident, the symptoms, and a physical examination, and is confirmed by x-rays and the withdrawal of air or blood from the thoracic cavity.

TREATMENT   In pneumothorax the free air can be withdrawn from the thoracic cavity with a syringe. If air continues to fill the cavity, surgical repair of the injury will be essential. In hemothorax, the hemorrhage will have to be controlled and this usually involves surgery. A diaphragmatic hernia will also require immediate surgical repair if compression of the heart and lungs is evident.

Drowning

Drowning is unusual in dogs since most are excellent swimmers. but it does occur if a dog falls through ice or into a swimming pool and cannot get out.

Treatment involves holding the dog up by the hind legs to drain the water out of the trachea (windpipe) and lungs and open the airway, and then to start CPR (*see* Cardiopulmonary Resuscitation, earlier in this chapter.) If the heart is beating, only artificial respiration will be necessary. The dog should be dried and kept warm.

Most dogs are saved by quick action by the owner, and few require veterinary care unless complications arise following revival.

Choking

Choking is the interruption of respiration by obstruction. It is not a common problem in dogs because they have strong

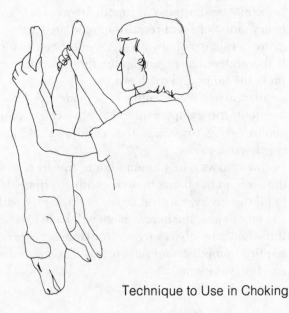

Technique to Use in Choking

cough reflexes and can usually dislodge obstructions readily. The most common cause of respiratory obstruction in dogs is bones.

SYMPTOMS   Sometimes there are no obvious signs of choking, but the dog will paw at the mouth, appear in distress, and lose consciousness if there is complete obstruction of the airway.

TREATMENT   The dog owner should open the dog's mouth and remove the obstruction if it is visible, while taking care not to get bitten if the dog is still conscious. Roll the dog's lips over its teeth to avoid a bite. If the object cannot be removed, hold the dog up by the hind legs and shake it vigorously while slapping it on the back.

If neither of these techniques succeeds in dislodging the obstruction or if the dog is too large to hold up, a Heimlich maneuver can be tried. Lay the dog on its stomach, straddle it and put the arms around the dog and clasp the hands to form a fist just below the dog's rib cage. Then apply a sudden, rapid upward movement with the clasped hands and repeat a few times. If this technique is too complicated, just lay the dog on its side and press forward and upwards just behind the rib cage a number of times.

If none of these efforts are successful, try to quickly reach a veterinarian or if this is not possible, as a last resort, perform a tracheotomy by cutting into the windpipe (trachea). The windpipe can be felt as a rigid tube in the front of the neck, and by opening it the dog's life can be saved. Any injuries to the area can be repaired later by a veterinarian. If the dog does not recover consciousness after an obstruction is dislodged, then apply CPR (*see* Cardiopulmonary Resuscitation, earlier in this chapter).

Status Epilepticus (*See also* Chapter 12, The Nervous System; Diseases and Disorders of the Brain: Epilepsy.)

Status epilepticus is repeated convulsions or seizures with no periods of consciousness between them. Emergency veterinary care is essential and involves the use of tranquilizers, sedatives, and even anesthetics to control the seizures. Supportive care and diagnostic tests to attempt to determine the cause will be necessary.

Poison*	Sources
Food	Garbage or spoiled foods
Carbamates	Insecticides
Organophosphates	Insecticides
Strychnine	Rodent poison or deliberate
Warfarin	Rodent poison
Snake venom	Venomous snakes
Chlorinated hydrocarbons	Insecticides
Arsenic	Rodent poison, insecticides, herbicides, ant poison, paint
Fungi	Cereal grains
Sodium fluoroacetate	Rodent and roach poisons
Thallium	Rodent, ant, and roach poisons
Metaldehyde	Snail bait
Toad toxin	*Bufo* species of toads
Lead	Old paint and plaster, lead weights and shot, lubricants, pesticides, leaded gasoline
Glycols	Antifreeze
Plant toxins	Poisonous plants
ANTU	Rodent poison
Acids	Car battery, cleaning agents
Alkalis	Cleaning/degreasing agents
Phenols	Carbolic acid and creosote
Zinc phosphide	Rat poison
Mercury	Disinfectants, antiseptics, pesticides, fungicides
Phosphorus	Rat and roach poisons

* In order of frequency encountered.

Poisoning

The preceding chart lists, in descending order of frequency, the poisons most often encountered in dogs today and the sources of these poisons.

SYMPTOMS   The signs and symptoms of most poisonings in dogs are quite similar, so it is not possible, in most cases, to make a diagnosis from them. The following chart lists the onset times—which depend on dosage as well as specific poison—and the symptoms of the most frequently encountered poisons in dogs. The poisons are grouped by type. (For sources of these poisons, *see* preceding chart.)

DIAGNOSIS   Poisoning in dogs can be from eating a poison or from absorbing it through the skin or the lungs. If the dog was exposed to or seen eating a poison, then there is no problem in diagnosis—if the symptoms are typical of poisoning from the poison involved. Otherwise, diagnosis is made from the history, clinical signs and symptoms, and a physical examination. It is difficult, except in a few poisons where the signs are very specific, to make a positive diagnosis of poisoning because the signs and symptoms are very similar in many poisonings, and the same signs are also seen in many other diseases. However, veterinary practitioners become experienced in identifying poison cases from the history and clinical signs, particularly those types of poisonings which are frequently encountered in their areas.

NOTE: At the University of Illinois there has been an Animal Toxicology Hotline since 1978. The number is (217) 333-3611. The service is available without charge twenty-four hours a day, seven days a week, and offers diagnostic assistance to veterinarians, agricultural workers, farmers, and animal owners in poisoning cases.

TREATMENT   All poisonings in dogs, except minor food poisonings and some chronic poisonings, are emergency situations and require immediate treatment. The chances of saving a poisoned dog are directly affected by how quickly

Specific Poisons and Symptoms

Poison	Onset Time and Symptoms
	RODENTICIDES
ANTU	4–6 hours. Vomiting, salivation, fluid in lungs, respiratory failure.
Sodium fluoroacetate	4–10 hours. Restless, urinates/defecates excessively, convulsions.
Strychnine	¼–2 hours. Restless, convulsions, respiratory arrest.
Thallium	Acute: within 24 hours. Vomiting, diarrhea, shortness of breath, paralysis, convulsions. Chronic: days to weeks. Poor appetite, hair loss, dry skin.
Warfarin	Slow hemorrhaging. Sudden death from internal bleeding or anemia, bloody feces, bloody mouth discharges, weakness, coma.
Zinc phosphide	¼–1 hour. Abdominal pain, vomiting, lethargy, coma.
Phosphorus	Immediate. Garlic odor to breath, vomiting, burns mouth and throat. Some dogs appear to recover, but in a few days relapse with liver and kidney damage, convulsions, coma.
	PESTICIDES
Arsenic	1–3 hours. Restless, vomiting, pain in abdomen, diarrhea, collapse.
Chlorinated hydrocarbons	1–2 hours. Can be absorbed through skin. Excitement, muscle tremors, salivation, convulsions; then depression, respiratory paralysis.
Organophosphates and Carbamates	1–2 hours. Most can be absorbed through skin. Salivation, vomiting, diarrhea, shortness of breath, contracted pupils, muscle tremors, depression, respiratory arrest.
Metaldehyde	1–12 hours. Incoordination, muscle tremors, frothing at mouth, loss of consciousness.

Specific Poisons and Symptoms (*continued*)

Poison	Onset Time and Symptoms
	GLYCOL
Antifreeze	½–1 hour. Trembling, vomiting, convulsions, coma. If survive, kidney failure develops.
	HEAVY METALS
Lead	Acute: days to weeks. Loss of appetite, vomiting, diarrhea, abdominal pain, vicious, champing jaws, frothing at mouth, blindness, convulsions, limb paralysis.
	Chronic: months. Loss of appetite and weight, depression, weakness, grinding teeth.
Mercury	Hours to days. Vomiting, diarrhea, salivation, paralysis, convulsions. Can be chronic development over weeks.
	OTHER
Acids & Alkalis	Immediate. Mouth and throat burns, thirst, abdominal pain, vomiting.
Phenols	½–2 hours. If concentrated, mouth and throat burns. Incoordination, depression, coma.
Food	1–24 hours. Nausea, vomiting, diarrhea, fever.

treatment is obtained; whether or not the poison is identified; how much was ingested or absorbed; how lethal the poison is; how fast-acting the poison is; and the dog's age and physical condition.

The emergency treatment for poisoning in dogs depends on whether the poison is corrosive or noncorrosive. Initial home treatment should only be done if the dog is seen taking the poison or known to have been exposed to a poison. If the dog is convulsing or comatose, do not try to treat, but rush it to the veterinary hospital. In *all* cases of poisoning, the earlier the treatment is started, the better the chance of saving the dog, so dog owners should not take time attempting home treatments if they have access to veterinary care.

Corrosive poisons. Corrosive poisons include all acids, most often from car batteries and cleaning agents; and alkalis such as lye, oven cleaner, and petroleum products in paint solvents and floor waxes. Phenols are also corrosive agents, commonly found in disinfectants, wood preservatives, fungicides, herbicides, and photographic developers.

Do not induce vomiting with corrosive poisons, because these agents burn the mouth, throat, and esophagus, and vomiting may increase the damage to these areas. If the dog owner sees the dog ingest such a product, the mouth should be flushed out with a hose, keeping the dog's head down to prevent choking. Also, rinse well any area of the skin that has contacted the poison. Then give the dog beaten-up egg whites, one per twenty pounds of body weight. To do this, tilt the dog's head up, hold the jaws closed, pull out the lower lip as a pouch and pour in a small amount of egg white, and allow the dog to swallow while rubbing the throat to stimulate swallowing (*see* Chapter 18, Home Medical Care; Administering Medications and Force-feeding: Liquid Medication). Repeat this until the dosage is complete. Take the dog and the poison container to the veterinary hospital as soon as possible.

Noncorrosive poisons. Most other poisons are noncorrosive. Vomiting should be induced immediately if the dog owner knows the dog has ingested poison, by giving one teaspoonful of 3% hydrogen peroxide per ten pounds of body weight, by mouth, using the method described above for egg whites. Repeat in ten minutes if the dog does not vomit, for two more times. If there is no hydrogen peroxide in the house, try putting one teaspoon of salt on the back of the dog's tongue as this will usually induce vomiting. A tablespoon of dry mustard in a cup of water will also induce vomiting. However, if veterinary care is readily available, do not delay. Bring the poison container and any vomitus to the veterinary hospital, as these may be helpful in making a diagnosis and in the choice of treatments.

Insecticide poisons. The most common and serious cause

of poisoning in dogs today is from the use of insecticides, mostly those used for flea control. Some dogs are overly sensitive to these agents and in other instances the dog owner does not use them according to directions. Most insecticides can be absorbed through the skin or the lungs and do not have to be ingested to cause poisoning. Immediate hosing down and bathing will reduce the amount of poison absorbed, once symptoms are noticed; but even if the dog appears to recover, see your veterinarian, as relapses and delayed symptoms are not unusual in insecticide poisonings.

Food poisons: (*See* Chapter 10, The Digestive System; Stomach Diseases and Disorders: Vomiting; *see also* same chapter; Intestinal Diseases and Disorders: Diarrhea.)

Inhaled poisons. Inhaled poisons, such as carbon monoxide from automobile exhaust, are absorbed through the lungs. If the dog is unconscious, the dog owner should give cardiopulmonary resuscitation (*see* earlier in this chapter), but should not delay in seeking veterinary treatment.

If the dog owner does not know if something the dog ate or was exposed to is a poison, or what type of poison it is, a veterinarian or poison control center should be called for advice.

Veterinary care. When bringing a poisoned dog to a veterinary hospital, let the receptionist or animal technician know at once that this is an emergency—do not politely wait to see the veterinarian! Veterinary treatment of poisoning includes some or all of the following:

1. Examination of the dog and the establishment of cardiac or pulmonary resuscitation if required to stabilize vital signs.

2. Induction of vomiting, except in unconscious dogs, or dogs which have ingested acids, alkalis, or petroleum products, or if the time since ingestion has been too long for this to be effective. Apomorphine, by injection, is the drug used most often to induce emesis (vomiting).

3. Prevention of further exposure to the poison by adminis-

tering activated charcoal to absorb the poison, gastric lavage (stomach pumping), laxatives, or an enema to dilute or remove the poison from the gastrointestinal tract.

4. Administration of an antidote, if available; not all poisons have known antidotes.

5. Aiding excretion and metabolism of the poison by using diuretics, intravenous fluids, and in some cases, dialysis.

6. Administration of pain relievers, if required, and sedatives or even anesthetics if convulsions are occurring.

Despite the best of medical care, not all poisoned dogs can be saved. Some dogs recover from the acute stages of poisoning, only to relapse in a few days because of liver and kidney damage.

POISONOUS ANIMALS AND INSECTS

Animals can be poisoned by bites from or contact with certain snakes, toads, salamanders, lizards, and insects. Such poisonings are relatively rare and few are fatal, particularly if treated.

Snakes

There are only four principal poisonous snakes in North America. These are divided into two types, pit vipers and coral snakes. The pit vipers are: rattlesnakes, in the Southwest and South; copperheads, in the East; and cottonmouths (water moccasins), in the South.

The bite of pit vipers leads to necrosis (tissue death) in the area of the bite, and if the venom dose is large, shock and other serious symptoms will eventually develop. Pit vipers can be identified by the pit between the eye and nostril; this is a sense organ to detect heat radiated by warm-blooded prey. Also, they have elliptical pupils, whereas most nonpoisonous North American snakes have round pupils. They have needle-like fangs, not found in nonvenomous snakes.

Coral snakes live in the southeastern part of the United States. Their venom poisons the nervous system and leads to heart and respiratory failure. The coral snake is usually less than three feet long and has red, yellow, and black rings, and a black head.

SYMPTOMS *Pit vipers.* Immediately following a bite from a pit viper there is some pain, and within ten minutes the area will swell and become reddened. The pain increases in severity as the area swells. The fang marks, often only one, are obvious at this stage, but may be obliterated after severe swelling occurs. Depending on the amount of venom injected and the size of the dog, salivation, vomiting, shortness of breath, and convulsions occur in a few hours; these lead eventually to shock, collapse, and without treatment, death. If the dog survives, and many do even without treatment, the tissue in the area of the bite dies and in time sloughs off (falls away), but this process may be complicated by infection.

Coral snakes. Bites from coral snakes do not cause as much pain or swelling as pit vipers, but signs of weakness, difficulty in breathing, heart irregularities, and shock develop in a few hours, and may lead to death.

Other snakes. Very often a dog is bitten by a nonpoisonous snake or a poisonous snake which did not inject any venom. In such instances, there is minimum pain and swelling, and none of the more serious signs described above develop. In these cases, cleaning the wound with 3% hydrogen peroxide and an antiseptic should be all that is necessary.

TREATMENT *Immediate care.* If bitten by a poisonous snake, a dog should be restrained, because the venom will spread more rapidly throughout the body if it runs around. Also, the snake should be identified, without, of course, inviting injury. An ice pack, if available, should be applied to the swelling. If the bite is on the limb, a *loose* tourniquet should be applied above the bite (you should be able to insert one finger easily beneath the tourniquet), which should not be released for one hour, by which time the dog should have been taken to a veterinarian. If veterinary care is not available, straight cuts can be made over the fang marks and the venom can be squeezed and sucked out by using a snakebite kit suction device, or by mouth. The latter poses some hazard to the person and should only be done in extreme emergencies and by someone who is informed on the technique.

Veterinary care. The veterinarian will administer antivenin (an antitoxin to venom), antibiotics, pain relievers, and in the case of pit viper bites, will suction and surgically remove the fang wound's area. In serious cases, supportive care and treatment for shock will be necessary. Fortunately, most dogs recover if treatment is not delayed.

PREVENTION People who plan on traveling with their dog in snake-infested areas far from veterinary services, should ask their veterinarian to supply them with antivenin, a snakebite kit, and instructions on how to handle such an emergency.

Toads

All toads secrete substances from skin glands that repulse animals, but most are not poisonous. The secretions of toads of the *Bufo* species, located in the Southeast, South, and Southwest, are poisonous to dogs which mouth them.

SYMPTOMS Symptoms occur immediately and include profuse salivation, vomiting and diarrhea, difficulty in breathing, heart irregularities, and convulsions. Some species produce very potent toxins and can kill a dog in fifteen minutes, but most, fortunately, are not serious hazards, and the dog recovers in a few hours. The highest mortality rate has been reported in Florida.

TREATMENT The dog's mouth should immediately be flushed with running water for a few minutes. If the dog's condition quickly worsens, emergency veterinary care is essential to save its life. Although there is no antidote, supportive and symptomatic care can save many dogs.

Salamanders

Some species of salamanders secrete a poison in their saliva.

SYMPTOMS If a dog is bitten by a poisonous salamander, signs of poisoning, which include salivation, muscle weakness, incoordination, vomiting, diarrhea, and convulsions, may develop. Most dogs are not seriously affected and very few die.

TREATMENT The dog's mouth should be washed out, and if severe symptoms develop, veterinary care should be sought.

Lizards

There are two poisonous lizards in the southwestern United States: Gila monsters and Mexican beaded lizards. These lizards have venom glands in their upper teeth.

SYMPTOMS Fortunately, lizards are not very aggressive, but if a dog is bitten, signs of pain, swelling, shock, and convulsions may develop.

TREATMENT Treatment is supportive and veterinary care is recommended. Work is being done on the development of an antivenin.

Insects and Other Stinging Pests

With the exception of bites from black widow spiders, poisonous insect bites or stings, such as those from tarantulas, bees, wasps, and scorpions, are not dangerous to dogs, although they can be painful. Application of ice cubes is usually all that is necessary, and, of course, if a stinger is seen, it should be removed. In rare cases, a dog will have a serious allergic reaction, and in these instances, veterinary care will be required. Black widow spider venom is fifteen times as potent as that of rattlesnakes. The symptoms are similar. A specific antivenin is available.

POISONOUS PLANTS

With the increasing popularity of house plants, the incidence of poisoning in dogs from toxic plants has been increasing.

The most common house plants of which all parts are poisonous, listed in alphabetical order, are:

- Azalea
- Bleeding Heart
- Boxwood
- Castor Bean
- Christmas Rose
- Crocus
- Daphne
- Delphinium
- Dieffenbachia
- Dumbcane
- Elephant Ear
- English Holly
- English Ivy
- Four-O'clock
- Foxglove
- Hydrangea
- Iris
- Jerusalem Cherry
- Larkspur
- Lily-of-the-Valley
- Laurel
- Monkshood
- Mountain Laurel
- Oleander
- Philodendron
- Poinsettia*
- Rhododendron
- Star of Bethlehem
- Yellow Jasmine
- Yew

Common house plants of which some parts are poisonous (the poisonous part follows listing in parentheses) are:

- Daffodil (bulb)
- Golden Chain (seeds)
- Hyacinth (bulb)

* The Society of American Florists claims that the toxicity information on poinsettia and mistletoe is misleading. Toxicity studies have been conducted on the poinsettia plant which indicated large quantities would have to be eaten even to cause even nausea and vomiting; these plants are also very bitter, so are unlikely to be eaten by dogs. The Consumer Product Safety Commission no longer requires caution labels on poinsettia plants. Mistletoe berries are poisonous, but are also very bitter and unlikely to be ingested under normal circumstances.

- Lantana (berries)
- Mistletoe (berries)*
- Morning Glory (seeds)
- Narcissus (bulb)
- Pine Tree (needles)
- Sweet Pea (seeds)

These are by no means exhaustive lists of plants with poisonous capabilities, so if a dog owner brings home a plant about which there is doubt, it should be checked with a nursery, poison control center, or the U.S. Department of Agriculture in their area.

Other sources of plant poisonings in dogs are grain contaminants, such as certain fungi, herbicides, and insecticides. Grains are used in commercial dog foods, which must meet government safety standards, so this type of poisoning is very rare today. Blue-green freshwater algae and mushrooms occasionally cause poisoning in dogs.

UNUSUAL DRUG POISONINGS

Some accidental, and occasionally deliberate, poisonings in dogs involve the following drugs:

Marijuana. Veterinarians are reporting cases of dogs under the influence of marijuana more frequently. Signs of depression, incoordination, and sleepiness are seen, but in high dosages severe depression can occur and hospital treatment may be required. Most cases are the result of dogs ingesting the owner's "pot" by accident, although in some cases the dogs have been deliberately fed the plant, for the amusement of the owners. The owner sometimes needs treatment more than the dog does in such instances!

Nicotine. Poisoning from nicotine is most often seen in puppies which have eaten cigarettes or cigars. Nicotine is a

* *See note opposite.*

stimulant, and salivation, vomiting, diarrhea, excitement, muscle tremors, and seizures may result from ingestion. If symptoms are severe, veterinary care is needed, as nicotine can be fatal.

Amphetamine. These cases of poisoning usually occur when dogs accidentally ingest the owner's appetite control tablets or sometimes illicit supplies. These are powerful stimulants and can lead to convulsions in high dosages, so treatment is essential if signs of poisoning are obvious.

Caffeine. This drug is also a strong stimulant and if caffeine-containing tablets are ingested by a dog, emergency veterinary care is essential. Fatalities are not unusual from caffeine overdosage.

17
Drugs

VETERINARY DRUGS

Veterinary drugs are the same as those used in human medicine, formulated specifically for animals according to the requirements of the individual species for which they are intended.

Drugs may be known by a number of different names—chemical, generic, and trade names. A chemical name is based on the chemical formula, e.g., 4-butyl-1, 2-diphenyl-3, 5-pyrazolidinedione. A generic, or nonproprietary, name is a drug name not protected by a trademark, e.g., for the same drug above: phenylbutazone. A trade, brand, or proprietary name is a drug name registered by a company which then becomes its exclusive property, e.g., for the above drug: Butatron (Osborn), Butazolidin (Jensen-Salsbery), Robizone-V (Robins).

There are thousands of drugs available for treating human and animal diseases and disorders. The following chart lists some of the major veterinary drug categories, and a few of the commonly used drugs in each category.

Quality and Cost

The general public and even many dog owners seem to think that veterinary drugs, such as antibiotics and vaccines, are lower in quality than those used for humans. There is no such thing as a "cheap" antibiotic or vaccine for pet or human. Exactly the same laboratory formulations and methods must

Veterinary Drugs

Drug Category	Generic Drug Name	Trade or Brand Name
Allergy	Methylprednisolone	Medrol
	Triamcinolone	Vetalog
	Dexamethasone	Azium
	Prednisone	Meticorten
Analgesics (Pain Relievers)	Aspirin	
	Acetaminophen	Tylenol
	Codeine	
	Morphine	
Anesthetics		
Intramuscular	Ketamine	Ketaset
Intravenous	Pentobarbital sodium	Nembutal
	Sodium thiopental	Pentothal
	Thiamylal sodium	Surital
Inhalation (Gas)	Methoxyflurane	Metofane
	Halothane	Fluothane
Local & Topical	Lidocaine	Xylocaine
Antacids	Magnesium hydroxide	Milk of Magnesia
	Aluminum/ Magnesium hydroxide and simethicone	Mylanta Maalox
Antiobiotics	(*See* Antimicrobials, later in this chapter)	
Anticoagulants	Heparin	
Anticonvulsants	Phenytoin	Dilantin
	Primidone	Anadone
Antidiarrheals	Kaolin and Pectin	Kaopectate
	Methscopolamine	Biosol
	Aminopentamide	Centrine
Antidotes	Charcoal, activated	
	Atropine	
	Nalorphine	Nalline
Antiemetics (Motion Sickness)	Chlorpromazine	Thorazine
	Piperacetazine	Psymod
	Prochlorperazine and Isopropamide	Darbazine
Antifungals	(*See* Antimicrobials, later in this chapter)	

Veterinary Drugs (*continued*)

Drug Category	Generic Drug Name	Trade or Brand Name
Antihistamines	Chlorpheniramine	Metrevet
	Tripelennamine	Re-Covr
	Diphenhydramine	Benadryl
Anti-inflammatories	(*See also* Corticosteroids, later in this chapter)	
	Phenylbutazone	Butazolidin
Antimicrobials	(*See* Antimicrobials, later in this chapter)	
Antiseptics	(*See* Antimicrobials, later in this chapter)	
Antispasmodics (Smooth Muscle Spasm Relief)	Atropine	
	Aminopentamide	Centrine
Antitussives (Inhibit Cough)	Trimeprazine	Temaril-P
	Multidrugs	Anti-Tuss
Biologicals	Vaccines (*See* Chapter 14, Infectious, Respiratory, and Hormonal Diseases; Vaccinations)	
Cancer Drugs	Nitrogen mustard	Mustargen
	Vincristine	Oncovin
	Cytarabine	Cytosar
	Hormone drugs	
Cardiovascular Agents	Digitalis	Digoxin
	Isoproterenol	Isuprel
Corticosteroids	(*See* Corticosteroids, later in this chapter)	
Dermatology Agents	(Multiple combination drugs for injectable, oral, and topical use with corticosteroids, antibiotics, and other agents)	
Dietary Supplements	Vitamins	
	Minerals	
	Special Diets	
	Milk Replacers	
Digestive Aids	Digestive enzymes	
Diuretics	Furosemide	Lasix
	Chlorothiazide	Diuril
Ear Preparations	(Ointments and solutions with corticosteroids, antibiotics, insecticides, and other agents)	
Emetics	Apomorphine	
	Ipecac	
Enzyme Preparations	Chymotrypsin	
	Streptokinase	

Veterinary Drugs (*continued*)

Drug Category	Generic Drug Name	Trade or Brand Name
Estrus Suppression (Birth Control)	Mibolerone Megestrol	Cheque Drops Ovaban
Eye Preparations	(Ointments and solutions with corticosteroids, antibiotics, atropine, and other agents)	
Hormones	Diethylstilbestrol Testosterone Insulin Thyroid Corticosteroids	
Insecticides		
External Use	Methylcarbamate Pyrethrins Rotenone	Carbaryl
Internal Use	Cythioate	Proban
Laxatives	Magnesium hydroxide Mineral oil Petrolatum	Milk of Magnesia Laxatone
Muscle Relaxants	Methocarbamol Xylazine	Robaxin Rompun
Musculoskeletal Disorders	Corticosteroids Phenylbutazone	Butazolidin
Nitrofurans	(*See* Antimicrobials, later in this chapter)	
Sedatives	Pentobarbital sodium Piperacetazine Xylazine	Nembutal Psymod Rompun
Solutions	Dextrose Electrolytes	
Sulfonamides	(*See* Antimicrobials, later in this chapter)	
Tranquilizers	Acetylpromazine Diazepam Chlorpromazine Piperacetazine Propiopromazine Trimeprazine Meprobamate	Acepromazine Valium Thorazine Psymod Tranvet Temaril Miltown
Urinary Acidifiers	Ammonium chloride Methionine	

Veterinary Drugs (*continued*)

Drug Category	Generic Drug Name	Trade or Brand Name
Worming Agents		
Roundworms	Piperazine	Pipcide
Round-, Hook- and Whipworms	Dichlorvos	Task
Tapeworms	Bunamidine	Scolaban
	Niclosamide	Yomesan
	Praziquantel	Droncit
Heartworms	Thiacetarsamide	Caparsolate
	Diethylcarbamazine	Caricide

be used to produce drugs and biologicals (vaccines) for veterinary or human medical use. All drugs are used first in laboratory animals to test their effects and potencies, prior to approval by the Food and Drug Administration for use in domestic animals, pets, or humans. The only real difference between human and veterinary drugs is in the strength of the drug, since dosage is related to body weight.

However, veterinary drugs for pets are not as expensive as human drugs for a number of reasons, none of which are related to quality: Since most pets weigh less than humans, less of the drug is needed; veterinarians dispense directly to their clients, thereby eliminating the extra cost of having a prescription filled by a pharmacist; veterinarians dispense drugs to their clients as a service and not for profit, so the mark-up on veterinary drugs is minimal; drug manufacturers often charge less for a veterinary drug than the same human drug because the overhead costs of packaging and distribution are less; and veterinarians use generic drugs wherever possible to minimize cost to their clients.

However, if a veterinarian writes a prescription and a dog owner has it filled by a pharmacy, the cost will be the same as for the equivalent prescription written by an MD.

Side Effects

The ideal drug cures the disease or disorder, or relieves the symptoms, without hurting the human or animal. Unfortunately, there is no such thing as an ideal drug. All drugs have undesirable side effects, some very hazardous. Therefore, it is important not to administer any drugs unless the benefits outweigh the risks involved. An accurate diagnosis should be obtained if possible before any drugs are administered, particularly if the more potent drugs need to be used on a long term basis.

SERIOUS SIDE EFFECTS   The more serious drug-related side effects are, fortunately, relatively rare, but do occur on occasion. Some of these are:

- Gastrointestinal hemorrhage and peptic ulcers, from corticosteroids, aspirin, and anticoagulants.
- Hemorrhages, from anticoagulants.
- Liver damage, from the tranquilizer chlorpromazine.
- Nervous system damage, from some antibiotics.
- Aplastic anemia, from chloramphenicol and phenylbutazone.
- Kidney failure, from some pain reliever drugs and antibiotics.
- Fetal development abnormalities, from many drugs.
- Infection and poor wound healing, from lowered immunity due to corticosteroids.
- Anaphylaxis, a serious allergic reaction, which can be fatal, from penicillin and antiserums.
- Carcinogenesis, cancer-producing effect of certain drugs.

LESS SERIOUS SIDE EFFECTS   Less serious drug-related side effects can cause damage, usually readily reversible, to the following organs or body systems:

- Skin—rashes, eruptions, itching.
- Blood—reversible anemias, blood coagulation disorders.
- Liver—abnormal function.

- Kidneys—damage to kidney cells.
- Nervous system—depression or stimulation, muscle tremors.
- Heart and blood vessels—arrhythmias and impaired circulation.
- Lungs—fluid buildup, hay fever, or asthma-like reactions.
- Gastrointestinal tract—nausea, vomiting, diarrhea.
- Endocrine system—depressed function of glands.
- Reproductive system—infertility.

Other side effects are interference with absorption of vitamins, minerals, and other nutrients; "sterile gut," a condition that results from long-term use of antibiotics or sulfonamides, which destroy the normal and necessary organisms in the gut, leading to digestive upsets and poor absorption of nutrients; chemical castration from excessive use of sex hormones; interference with electrolyte balance; suppression of function of the adrenal glands; abnormal oxygenation of tissues; and fever.

Antimicrobials

Antimicrobials are any drugs which can be used in humans or animals to kill or inhibit multiplication of microbes or microorganisms (bacteria, viruses, fungi) causing disease. These drugs act by interfering with the organisms' growth or reproduction. Antimicrobials include antiseptics, antibiotics, sulfonamides, nitrofurans, and antifungal and antiviral drugs. These drugs are derived from bacteria or molds, or made from chemical synthesis.

All antimicrobials are potent drugs, and proper usage is important to avoid serious side effects. Before using any antimicrobial agents, the seriousness of the illness, the toxicity of the drug of choice, the animal's age and condition, the danger of an allergic reaction, the side effects, and the cost must be taken into account. An accurate diagnosis of the disease and identification of the organism, if possible, must also

302 Drugs

be made. Culture of the organism and sensitivity testing is necessary to determine which antimicrobials will be effective in treatment. It goes almost without saying that the correct dosage and an adequate time of treatment are important, as is careful monitoring for serious side effects. Early treatment will allow time for use of another drug if the first choice is not effective, or if there are serious side effects.

Many organisms have become resistant to antimicrobials due to improper usage, particularly inadequate dosing for too short a period of time. It should also be emphasized that antibiotics are not effective against viruses and should only be used in viral infections if the possibility of secondary bacterial infection is present.

The following chart lists the most frequently used antimicrobials.

Corticosteroids

There are two types of natural corticosteroid hormones produced by the adrenal glands: *glucocorticosteroids,* which have anti-inflammatory effects and also influence carbohydrate, fat, and protein metabolism; and *mineralocorticosteroids,* which regulate the electrolytes such as sodium and potassium, and the water balance in the body.

Synthetic corticosteroids are man-made drugs and their effects are similar to natural corticosteroid hormones. They are used mainly for their anti-inflammatory effect or to treat severe body stress, such as shock, and in serious diseases.

Corticosteroid drugs were first developed for medical use in the 1950s, and there are now over fifty of them. The most commonly used in veterinary medicine are (generic names): cortisone, hydrocortisone, prednisone, prednisolone, methylprednisolone, triamicinolone, dexamethasone, bethamethasone, fludrocortisone, fluoroprednisolone, flumethasone, and fluocinolone.

Corticosteroid drugs are not curative, but are used to reduce or alleviate symptoms in many diseases and disorders, such as in skin diseases—especially those of allergic origin; respiratory diseases—chronic or allergic; adrenal gland malfunction; shock; colitis; musculoskeletal diseases and disorders, such as arthritis and bursitis; eye diseases; diseases of the immune system; and cancer.

Antimicrobial Agents

Antiseptics	Antibiotics	Sulfonamides
Lysol	Penicillins	Sulfamerazine
pHisoHex	Streptomycin	Sulfamethazine
Zephiran	Chloramphenicol	Sulfadimethoxine
Iodine	Tetracyclines	Sulfanilamide
Betadine	Erythromycin	Sulfathiazole
3% Hydrogen Peroxide	Lincomycin	Sulfadiazine
	Gentamicin	Sulfapyridine
Mercurochrome	Kanamycin	Sulfamethizole
Merthiolate	Neomycin	Sulfacetamide
	Tylosin	Sulfisoxazole
	Spectinomycin	Sulfaguanidine
	Cephalosporins	Sulfaquinoxaline
	Novobiocin	Sulfachlorpyridazine
	Bacitracin	Sulfabromomethazine
	Polymyxin B	Sulfamethoxypyridazine

Nitrofurans	Antifungals	Antivirals*
Nitrofurantoin	Griseofulvin	Idoxuridine
Nitrofurazone	Amphotericin B	Cytarabine
Nifuraldezone	Nystatin	Trifluridine
Furazolidone		Acyclovir

* There are few antiviral agents available for use; those that have been developed are for limited, special-purpose uses. The reason there has been little development of antiviral agents for use in humans or animals is that the agents that block viral growth also block normal cell growth. Many antiviral agents have been developed in research, but most are too toxic to give to patients.

UNDESIRABLE EFFECTS Corticosteroids are used for long periods in dogs, most commonly to treat allergic skin diseases. Their anti-inflammatory, anti-allergic actions give quick relief to the itching, scratching dog. It is this long-term use that leads to the undesirable side effects. Short-term use, even in very high doses, such as are appropriate for shock, seldom causes serious problems. These drugs are also immunosuppressive (they depress the immune system), which results in an increased susceptibility to infection. Excessive usage or too-sudden withdrawal can lead to problems.

Excessive Usage. Long-term (more than four months) use, or high dosages, may result in signs of a condition called Cushing's syndrome, due to the presence of too much synthetic adrenal hormones in the body. The early signs are excessive thirst and urination, loss of hair, darkening of skin color, and a thin dog with an enlarged, pendulous abdomen. Later in this syndrome, lethargy, weakness, bone pain, bone fractures, poor wound healing, easy bruising, and liver problems occur.

Too-Sudden Withdrawal. Corticosteroid drugs suppress the natural function of the adrenal glands. Therefore, if corticosteroid drugs are stopped suddenly or the body requires extra adrenal hormones because of stress, the adrenal glands may not be able to start working again fast enough to produce adequate quantities of the hormones, and the dog can go into a life-threatening adrenal shock or crisis, also called an Addisonian crisis. Early signs of this are lethargy, depression, fatigue, weakness, vomiting, diarrhea, loss of appetite, and weight loss. In a short period (less than twenty-four hours), in severe cases, convulsions, coma, and death will occur.

PROPER LONG-TERM USE OF CORTICOSTEROIDS Like antibiotics, corticosteroids have been overused and abused for many years, particularly in the treatment of skin problems in dogs. However, long-term corticosteroid use is necessary in certain cases; the key to safe use is skilled clinical management. If the following guidelines are adhered to, few and usually no harmful side effects will occur, even in dogs that have to stay on these drugs for years:

1. Use only oral corticosteroids, such as prednisone, prednisolone, or methylprednisolone, because dosage can be easily adjusted. Long-acting injections should only be used in hard-to-treat dogs, or in severe cases.

2. A high initial dose (induction dose) for up to one week may be required, but this should be reduced weekly until the smallest dose which will control the symptoms has been reached. This is called the maintenance dose.

3. Use alternate-day treatment if possible to avoid continuous depression of adrenal gland function. This gives the adrenal glands a chance to recover on nontreatment days.

4. Give the drug in the morning when natural adrenal secretion is highest. This gives the adrenal glands a chance to recover later in the day.

5. Use for short periods, less than three months, if possible.

6. Increase the dosage, under veterinary supervision, during periods of stress, such as travel, move to a new home, boarding, infection, injury, surgery, etc., to prevent adrenal shock, because the body requires extra adrenal hormones under such circumstances (*see* Too-Sudden Withdrawal).

7. When withdrawing treatment, gradually reduce the dosage over three to four weeks, but *never* abruptly stop this medication (*see* Too-Sudden Withdrawal). If a sudden stoppage is necessary, a veterinarian can give adrenal stimulating drugs to prevent an adrenal crisis.

8. Watch for early signs of overdosage such as excessive appetite, thirst, and urination; darkening of the skin; and weight gain (*see* Excessive Usage). Mildly increased appetite and drinking on the day of dosage is not unusual and of no significance.

9. Watch for early signs of adrenal gland suppression during stress or withdrawal, such as lethargy and weakness (*see* Too-Sudden Withdrawal).

Corticosteroids are still wonder drugs, but their potential to cause injurious side effects if improperly used is as great as is their effectiveness in treatment. They should only be used if no other treatment is available.

Aspirin for Dogs

Aspirin (acetylsalicylic acid) can be given to dogs, but care must be taken to give the correct dosage. Because of its availability and low cost, the value and potency of aspirin as a drug is underestimated by most people. Further, while many people think it is innocuous, in reality it can be very toxic and even lead to death if misused.

USES Aspirin relieves pain that arises from superficial wounds, and from inflamed joints, tendons, and muscles. It also reduces inflammation (hot, painful swellings). It decreases the temperature in fever, but has no effect on normal body temperature. Aspirin does not help relieve the pain from internal organs. Aspirin is an inexpensive and safe drug when used properly, and can be given by dog owners to their dogs, on occasion, for muscular and joint pain, for pain following surgery, for head and dental pain, or to help reduce a fever.

DOSAGE FOR DOGS Aspirin is absorbed in the stomach and intestines of dogs, and eliminated (excreted) from the system in the urine.

The dosage for dogs is ¾ grain (48¾ milligrams) for every ten pounds of body weight every twelve hours. The dosage is lower than that used in humans because it takes dogs up to four times as long to break down and eliminate aspirin from their systems. Prolonged administration—that is, for more than a week—should only be done under veterinary supervision. Aspirin should not be used in puppies under two months of age or in pregnant dogs.

SIDE EFFECTS Overdosage, or an oversensitivity to aspirin in some dogs, can cause difficulty in breathing, vomiting, gastrointestinal bleeding, and anemia-like conditions.

Warning: Aspirin can be fatal to cats because cats excrete the drug very slowly, and this can lead to poisoning. For this reason, aspirin is not recommended for use in cats except under veterinary supervision.

Laetrile (*See* Chapter 15, Cancer; Laetrile and Cancer)

DMSO

Dimethyl sulfoxide, or DMSO, a by-product of the lumber industry, is discussed here because it has received a lot of exaggerated attention in the press and has been referred to as a wonder drug and "a healer of all kinds of human and animal ills."

USES   DMSO has been approved by the Food and Drug Administration (FDA), for over ten years, for use by veterinarians to reduce swelling and pain caused by trauma and diseases (usually musculoskeletal disorders) in horses and dogs. In humans, DMSO is approved for use to treat one disease only: interstitial cystitis, a bladder disorder. A black market DMSO is being used by many people to treat mostly muscle and joint pains.

DMSO is not a panacea, but it is useful because of its ability to penetrate the unbroken skin and to reduce inflammation and pain. It also improves circulation in the area of application. Because it can penetrate the skin, other drugs such as antibiotics and corticosteroids can be combined with it and carried to the site of inflammation.

SIDE EFFECTS   There are no well-documented cases of serious toxicity from the use of DMSO at present, but there may be in the future, particularly as a result of the use of black market products which may not be pure. All drugs have some side effects, and DMSO is no exception. These include skin irritation, garlic breath odor, nausea, diarrhea, and allergies. Heavy doses have caused eye problems in rabbits.

18

Home Medical Care

HOME MEDICINE CABINET

Most households have home medicine cabinets which contain a variety of over-the-counter (OTC) medications. Although these products were purchased and formulated for human use, most can be safely used in dogs on a first-aid basis. Adjustments will need to be made in the dosages on a weight basis for dogs. As a rough guide, the human adult dose can be used in dogs over one hundred pounds; the dose for children can be used in medium-sized dogs; and the infant dose can be used in small dogs or halved for toy breeds.

The following chart lists the drugs most commonly found in the home medicine cabinet and the indications for first-aid use in dogs. It is always best to obtain veterinary advice before using OTC drugs in dogs, but if this is not possible, then the drugs listed can be used on occasion. Their inclusion in this chart is not a recommendation for their use in dogs. Care must be taken in using OTC medications on the skin of dogs because of the danger of poisoning if the dog licks it off. If a dog has a bad reaction to any drug, veterinary or OTC, stop using it at once and check with your veterinarian.

Other useful home medicine cabinet items for use with dogs are: a rectal thermometer, which can be lubricated with petroleum jelly before insertion, to check a dog's temperature (normal is 101.5° Fahrenheit); bandages for wounds, and which are also useful to tie around the dog's nose and chin as

Home Medicine Cabinet Drugs

Drug Category	Indications for Use	Drug Name*
Analgesics	Pain relief	Aspirin (for dosage, *see* Chapter 17, Drugs; Aspirin for dogs) Tylenol
Antacids	Stomach upset	Di-Gel Mylanta Milk of Magnesia
Antibiotic Ointment	Minor wounds	Bacitracin Terramycin
Antidiarrheals	Diarrhea	Kaopectate Pepto-Bismol
Antiemetics	Nausea and vomiting Motion sickness	Pepto-Bismol Bonine Dramamine
Antiflatulents	Excess gas	Mylicon Mylanta
Antihistamines	Allergy, hay fever	Dristan Allerest
Antiseptics	Minor wounds	3% Hydrogen Peroxide Bactine Betadine Listerine Mercurochrome Merthiolate Campho-Phenique
Antitussives	Coughing	Vicks Formula 44 Robitussin
Bronchodilators	Asthma and hay fever	Bronkaid Primatene capsules
Ear Preparations	Cleaning ears	Mineral oil
Eye Preparations	Eye irritation	Murine Visine Artificial tears
Laxatives	Constipation	Milk of Magnesia (stimulant) Ducolax (stimulant) Mineral oil (lubricant) Dioctyl (stool softener)

Home Medicine Cabinet Drugs (*continued*)

Drug Category	Indications for Use	Drug Name*
		Metamucil (bulk laxative) Fleet enema
Poisoning	To induce vomiting	(*See* Chapter 16, Emergency Care; Emergency Cases: Poisoning, Treatment) 3% Hydrogen Peroxide Ipecac
Respiratory Disease Drugs	Minor upper and lower respiratory infections	Coricidin Dristan Contac Triaminicin Novahistine Sudafed Actifed
Skin Preparations	Skin diseases and disorders	Not advisable as there is danger of toxicity if dog licks medication off skin
Vitamins and Minerals	Deficiencies or supplements	Best to use those formulated for dogs

* Most are trade or brand names.

a muzzle; eye droppers (preferably plastic) for giving liquid medication; Q-Tips for cleaning the ears; sterile gauze pads for wounds or as pressure pads to stop bleeding; cotton; adhesive tape; ice packs; a heating pad; a magnifying glass; and instruments such as scissors, tweezers, etc.

SYMPTOMS OF ILLNESS

Although it is seldom possible to diagnose the cause of a dog's illness from the symptoms alone, the following symptoms reference chart may be helpful to the dog owner who is attempting to determine the cause of an illness, and to decide whether to try home treatment or seek veterinary care.

Symptoms Reference Chart

Symptom	Cause
Abdomen, swelling	Stomach torsion; heart failure; liver disease; peritonitis; urethral blockage; abdominal tumors.
Abscess	Pus accumulation from infection in body organ or part.
Acne	Bacterial skin disease.
Anemia	External and internal bleeding; blood coagulation disorders; stomach ulcers; nutritional deficiencies; fleas; hookworms; blood parasites; poisons; cancer; immune system disorders; liver disease; kidney failure; infections; radiation sickness.
Appetite:	
Abnormal	Gastrointestinal disease; pancreatic disease; nutritional deficiencies; stool eating—cause unknown.
Increased	Tapeworms; hormone imbalances; diabetes mellitus.
Poor or none	Generalized and infectious diseases; heart disease; kidney disease; gastrointestinal disease; mouth inflammations; hormonal imbalances; pharyngitis; esophagitis; tonsillitis; advanced cancer.
Baldness	Skin disease; hormonal imbalances.
Bleeding	External or internal from injury or disease.
Blindness	Retinal disease; cataracts; glaucoma; central nervous system injury or disease.
Bloating	(*See* Abdomen, swelling)
Breasts, swollen	Infections; tumors.
Breath (bad)	Mouth inflammation; gum and tooth disease; digestive problems; kidney disease.
Breathing, abnormal	Respiratory disease; shock; heart failure; poisons; high fever; heat stroke; eclampsia (milk fever).
Choking	Foreign bodies, especially bones.
Circling	Inner ear disease; central nervous system disease.

Symptoms Reference Chart (*continued*)

Symptom	Cause
Constipation	Anal gland disease; low-bulk diet; excess bones; dry food with inadequate water; gastrointestinal or abdominal tumors; enlarged prostate; intestinal parasite blockage; foreign bodies; injury; inadequate exercise; obesity; old age; nervous system disease.
Convulsions (Seizures, Fits)	Central nervous system disease and injury; poisons; heat stroke; brain tumors; epilepsy; kidney failure; heart disease; parasites; lack of oxygen; following distemper; low blood sugar; electrocution; eclampsia (milk fever).
Coughing	Roundworms; heart failure; upper and lower respiratory disease; poisons; heartworms; asthma; distemper; parasites.
Deafness	Ear disease or injury; ear or brain tumors; following distemper; certain drugs; old age.
Dehydration	Inadequate water intake; vomiting; diarrhea; high fever; kidney failure.
Diarrhea (More serious if bloody)	Worms; food allergy; diabetes mellitus; kidney disease; liver disease; pancreatic disease; poisons; infectious diseases; gastrointestinal tumors; stomach torsion; foreign bodies; internal injuries; anal gland disease; food poisoning; intestinal infections; intestinal obstruction; defective intestinal absorption; nervous system diseases and injuries; shock; trauma.
Dislocations	Injury.
Drinking, excess	Heart disease; kidney failure; shock; hormonal imbalances; pancreatic disease; diabetes mellitus; cystitis; hot weather.
Drooling	Motion sickness; nausea; fear; injury; poisons; mouth inflammation; foreign body in mouth or throat; gum and tooth disease; stomach torsion; eclampsia (milk fever).
Ear discharge	Ear disease; foreign body; abscess; tumors.

Symptoms Reference Chart (*continued*)

Symptom	Cause
Eyes:	
Cloudy	Injury; corneal inflammation or ulcer; cataract; glaucoma; infection.
Discharge	Allergy; eye disease; infection; infectious diseases such as distemper; foreign body; irritants; injury; eye parasites; tumors; eyelid abnormalities; lack of tears; sinus infections; respiratory disease.
Dry	Dehydration; lack of tears.
Sunken	Dehydration; starvation.
Fever	Infections and inflammations.
Fits	(*see* Convulsions)
Flatulence (Gas)	Swallowing air; gas-producing foods; milk; high meat protein diets; rich carbohydrate diets; obesity; liver disease; pancreatic disease.
Gagging	Choking; vomiting attempts.
Gas	(*See* Faltulence)
Grass eating	Not known. Possibly need for fiber or other nutritional requirement. To induce vomiting.
Gums	
Bluish	Heart disease; respiratory disease.
Dry	Dehydration.
Pale	Anemia; shock; cancer; internal and external bleeding.
Red	Gum infection and inflammation; heat stroke.
Haircoat:	
Change or loss	Skin disease; allergy; mange; ringworm; hormonal imbalances.
Dull	Worms; skin disease; liver disease; kidney disease; malnutrition; low fat diet; hormonal imbalances.
Head shaking	Ear disease; fleas; ear mites; ear hematoma.
Head tilt	Middle ear infection; tumor; brain injury or disease.
Heart:	
Fast	Fever; shock; heart disease; heat stroke.
Irregular	Heart disease.

Symptoms Reference Chart (*continued*)

Symptom	Cause
Weak	Shock; heart disease
Hives	Allergy
Hoarseness	Laryngitis; excessive barking; respiratory infection; foreign body; irritants; tumor.
Itching	External parasites; allergy; skin disease; ear disease; liver disease.
Lameness (limping)	Injury; bone infection; nervous system disorders; dislocations; fractures; sprains; strains; abscesses; foreign bodies; hip dysplasia; arthritis.
Licking	Skin disease; wounds; discharges from anus, vagina, or prepuce.
Lumps	Tumors; abscesses; hives; hernias, hematomas.
Nausea	(*See* Vomiting)
Nose discharge	Respiratory infection; allergy; inhaled irritants; distemper; trauma; foreign body; tumors; tooth and sinus infections; nasal parasites.
Obesity	Overeating; hormonal imbalances.
Paralysis	Injury; poisons; ticks; rabies; brain and spinal cord diseases, disorders and injuries; intervertebral disc, eclampsia (milk fever); tumors.
Pulse	(*See* Heart)
Pupils:	
Constricted	Poisons; bright light.
Dilated	Poisons; darkness; central nervous system injury; eclampsia (milk fever); glaucoma; death.
Hazy	Cataracts; old age changes.
Respiration	(*See* Breathing)
Restlessness	Stomach torsion; nervous system diseases and disorders; eclampsia (milk fever); poisons; pain.
Salivation	(*See* Drooling)
Scooting, on bottom	Anal sac disease; tapeworm segments passing out of anus; anal disease.
Scratching	External parasites; skin disease; ear disease; boredom.
Seizures	(*See* Convulsions)
Shedding	(*See* Haircoat)

Symptoms Reference Chart (*continued*)

Symptom	Cause
Shivering	Scared; pain; fever; cold; excitement.
Shock	Anaphylaxis (severe allergic reaction); pancreatic disease; poisons; trauma; heart failure; advanced infections; dehydration; advanced cancers; peritonitis.
Skin:	
Darkening	Hormonal imbalances; acanthosis nigricans; chronic skin disease.
Greasy	Seborrhea and other skin diseases.
Scaly/dry	Skin disease; low fat diet; kidney disease.
Sores/scabs	Skin disease; injuries.
Sneezing	Allergy; rhinitis; sinusitis; foreign body in nose.
Snoring	Long soft palate (bulldogs); post-nasal drip from allergy.
Snorting	Allergy; food stuck in throat.
Stiffness	Arthritis; old age.
Stomach distension	Overeating; roundworms in pups; stomach torsion.
Swallowing, difficulty	Rabies; mouth diseases and disorders; esophageal diseases; foreign bodies.
Swelling	(*See* Lumps *and* Abdomen, swelling)
Teeth, discoloration	Severe disease; nutritional deficiency; parasites; and certain drugs during first two months of life.
Temperature:	
Increase	Infections and inflammations.
Low	Shock; puppies, before whelping; kidney failure; debilitating diseases; frostbite.
Thirst	(*See* Drinking, excess)
Twitching (muscle jerks)	Skin disease; external parasites; nervous system injury; following distemper; kidney failure; eclampsia (milk fever); poisons.
Unconsciousness	Injury; shock; poisons; heat stroke; central nervous system diseases and injuries; heart failure; diabetes mellitus; coma.
Urination:	
Bloody	Kidney disease; cystitis; poisons.
Decreased or difficult	Prostate disease or enlargement; urethral blockage; kidney disease; tumors.

Symptoms Reference Chart (*continued*)

Symptom	Cause
Dribbling	Hormonal imbalances especially older spayed female; prostate enlargement; bladder stones; partial urethral blockage; nervous system diseases and injury (spinal discs); tumors; trauma.
Increased	Kidney disease; cystitis; heart disease; hormonal imbalances; pancreatic disease; diabetes mellitus.
None	Advanced kidney disease; shock; trauma; nervous system injury; complete urethral blockage; bladder rupture.
Uterine discharge	Uterine diseases and disorders.
Vomiting	Overeating; bloat; worms; pharyngitis; tonsillitis; esophageal dilation; stomach ulcers; digestive problems; infectious diseases such as distemper; diabetes mellitus; poisons; heat stroke; motion sickness; food allergy or poisoning; intestinal obstruction; gastrointestinal tumors; shock; pancreatic disease; liver disease; kidney disease; nervous system diseases and disorders; trauma.
Weakness	Anemia; heart disease; hormonal imbalances; liver disease; pancreatic disease; generalized disease; worms; kidney failure; old age.
Weight loss	Worms; chronic diseases; kidney disease; pancreatic disease; liver disease; old age.
Wheezing	Allergy; asthma; emphysema; pneumonia.
Wounds	Injuries

TEMPERATURE, RESPIRATORY RATE, AND HEART RATE (PULSE)

Normal values for the dog are:

Temperature	101°–102° Fahrenheit (38.3°–38.8° Centigrade)
Heart Rate (Pulse)	70–100 beats per minute in large dogs; 90–120 beats per minute in small or young dogs
Respiratory Rate	10–30 breaths per minute.

Taking a Dog's Temperature

It is best to use a rectal thermometer when taking a dog's temperature, but an oral one can be used if a rectal one is not available. Shake the thermometer below 95° Fahrenheit and lubricate it with petroleum jelly, mineral oil, or even vegetable oil if that is all that is available. If possible, have the dog standing (*see* Restraining a Dog During Treatment, later in this chapter), raise the tail, and gently insert the thermometer through the anus and into the rectum to about one-half of the thermometer's length for the average-sized dog, less for small dogs. Never push hard. With gentle pressure, the dog will relax the muscles around the anus, and the thermometer will readily slide into the rectum. Leave the thermometer in place for at least two minutes, and do not let go of it or the dog may suck it into the rectum. Then remove it, wipe it clean, and read the temperature. Most dogs have a normal body temperature between 100° and 102° Fahrenheit, but if the dog is ex-

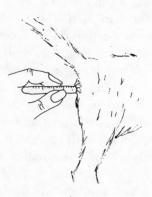

Method of Taking a Dog's Temperature

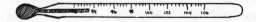

cited or upset, or if it is a very hot day, 103° Fahrenheit is not considered abnormal.

Measuring the Respiratory Rate in a Dog

Because dogs to not sweat through their skins, they must vaporize large volumes of water from their lungs to maintain normal body temperature. As a result, their respiratory rate varies considerably, depending on the environmental temperature and the amount of exertion. Therefore, to determine the normal respiratory rate, it needs to be measured with the dog in a resting state.

The chest movements can be readily counted in a dog lying quietly, and the normal range is ten to thirty breaths per minute. The inspiratory movement, when the dog is taking in air, is easier to measure than the expiratory, or expelling, of air movement. Another method is to hold a tissue, a light piece of cloth, or a feather in front of the dog's nose and count each time the object is pushed forward as the dog expires. A mirror can also be used and when placed in front of the dog's nose it will cloud up with each expiration; this latter method is useful to determine if an unconscious dog is breathing at all.

More significant than the rate of respiration in dogs is the breathing itself. Is it regular or irregular? Is the dog taking a normal breath, or breathing extra deeply or shallowly? Is the dog having any difficulty in breathing? If breathing is abnormal, it helps if the dog owner puts an ear to the dog's chest and listens for any fluid sounds (gurgles) in the lungs, which could indicate a developing respiratory infection or pneumonia, or in accident cases, chest cavity hemorrhage or pulmonary edema (fluid accumulation in the lungs).

Measuring the Heart Rate or Pulse in a Dog

To measure the heart rate, lay the dog on its right side. The heartbeat can be felt with the fingers or the palm of the hand placed on the chest just behind the dog's left elbow with the leg extended, or under the elbow with the leg adducted

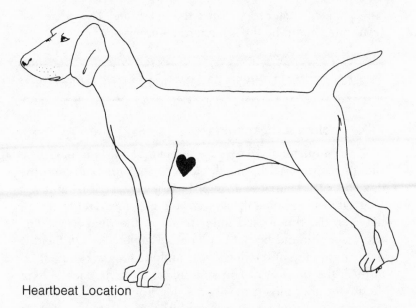

Heartbeat Location

(drawn toward the body). The actual position of the heart is in the lower part of the left chest cavity between the fifth and seventh ribs. If you put your ear to the dog's chest at this position, the heartbeat can readily be heard. The normal rate is between 70 and 120 beats per minute in the resting dog. Small and young dogs have faster rates than large adult dogs, and the rate increases with exercise and higher temperatures. There is a normal variation in the heart rhythm in resting dogs; the heart rate increases with inspiration and decreases with expiration. This is referred to technically as sinus arrhythmia. Sinus arrhythmia can also be associated with heart disease.

The femoral pulse is used to measure pulse rate in the dog. It is located on the inside of the rear leg between the knee and hip joint, close to where the leg joins the body. The pulse can be felt just in front of the femur bone and is more readily located and measured in the standing dog. Without practice, the femoral pulse can be difficult to locate in dogs, so it is much easier to measure the heart rate. The pulse and heart rate should be the same in the normal dog.

ADMINISTERING MEDICATIONS AND FORCE-FEEDING

Pills, Tablets, or Capsules

To administer a pill to a dog, the dog should preferably be standing. This will be much easier if someone can hold the dog so that it cannot squirm or back away (*see* Restraining a Dog During Treatment, later in this chapter). Hold the pill between the thumb and index finger of the right hand. The dog's head should be held up at a 45° angle. The left hand is put over the top of the dog's nose and the fingers can be used to push the dog's upper lips under its teeth on each side of the upper jaw. This prevents the dog from closing its mouth again or from biting, as it will not bite through its own lips. At the same time place the third, or middle, finger of the right hand on the front teeth of the lower jaw and pull downward to open the mouth further. Quickly insert the pill as far back on the tongue as possible, or in small dogs, drop it into the mouth. Remove the hand from the inside of the dog's mouth and close the mouth with the left or right hand around the jaws, while still keeping the head tilted up. Rub the front of the throat gently with the free hand to stimulate swallowing.

If this fails and the dog spits out the pill, try lubricating the pill with butter or oil to make it easier for the dog to swallow. However, this also has the disadvantage of making the pill harder to hold!

If the dog is still uncooperative, try hiding the pill in a food treat. It can also be crushed, or empty a capsule and mix it well with a small amount of a favorite food, but check with a veterinarian before doing this, as some medications have a special coating designed to be absorbed in the intestines and

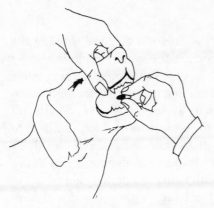

Administering Pills, Tablets, or Capsules

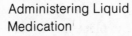

Administering Liquid Medication

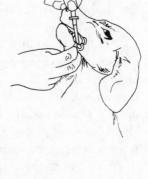

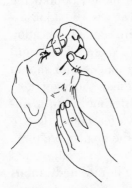

Rubbing Throat to Induce Swallowing

their effectiveness will be nullified if the coating is broken open. Unfortunately, most pills and tablets, when crushed, and most capsule contents, when emptied out, taste bad, so few dogs will be fooled more than once by this technique.

Dogs are not hard to medicate orally, but if there is difficulty, do contact a veterinarian, as there are many alternative methods of administering most medications. It is important that a dog receive the full course of prescribed medications.

Liquid Medication

Restraint, standing position, head angle, and rubbing the throat to stimulate swallowing are the same for administering liquid and pill medications. To give liquid medications, use a plastic (never glass because the dog may bite through it) graduated eye dropper or a small syringe with the needle removed. A spoon can be used, but it is much more difficult to work with. An assistant will be needed to hold the dog's mouth closed. Use one hand to pull out the dog's lips at the corner of one side of the mouth to make a pouch alongside the molar teeth, and use the other hand to place the liquid from the dropper in this area. Quickly close the lips and allow the dog to swallow.

Another technique is to place the liquid medication on the tongue by pushing the dropper into the mouth behind the large canine teeth. Liquid medications can also be administered much the same way as pills, by squirting the medication on the tongue while holding the mouth open. The liquid should not be placed too far back on the tongue, nor should too much be given at one time, or the dog may choke on it.

With any of these methods of administering liquid medications, do not give more than one or two teaspoons (five to ten milliliters), depending on the size of the dog, at one time. If the dose is larger than this, allow the dog to swallow and repeat until the full dose is given. Giving liquid medications to dogs can be a messy procedure, as they may spit it out, so choose a location that can be cleaned up easily.

Liquid medications can be added to the dog's food; many are designed to be given this way and are not at all distasteful to the dog. However, to be sure the dog receives the full dosage, mix the medications with a small amount of the dog's favorite food and make sure the dog eats it all.

Force-Feeding

Provided they are conscious, and are not vomiting or having diarrhea, dogs that do not eat may need to be force-fed. The veterinarian will recommend what to feed, depending on the nature of the illness, but most liquid diets for sick dogs will include some or all of the following ingredients: meat-type baby food, beaten-up egg yolks, meat or chicken soups, Karo syrup, and water to make the mixture of liquid consistency. Human liquid diets such as Ensure can be used for a few days if necessary.

The technique for force-feeding is the same as for liquid medication, but as a larger quantity will need to be given, a large plastic syringe or a kitchen baster is more convenient to use. It is very important not to give the dog more than it can swallow at one time. A sick dog should not be further stressed, so allow the dog to rest between each mouthful, and preferably give small feedings every few hours throughout the day rather than one or two large feedings.

A dog that is ill can often be coaxed into eating if the owner hand-feeds it with tasty food treats. Also, baby food can be smeared on the tongue, roof of the mouth, or even the lips and teeth, if the dog is still capable of licking it off and swallowing it. A dog that is not drinking will need to be given water as well.

Never try to force-feed a very depressed or an unconscious dog. Ill dogs should not be force-fed unless the veterinarian recommends it.

Ear Medicating

It is not difficult to medicate dogs' ears. Most ear medications are supplied as ointments in tubes with long nozzles, or as liquids in squirt bottles with pointed tips, to make it easy to place the medications into the external ear canal. Hold the tip of the ear flap or lobe straight up with the fingers of the left hand. Insert the medication container into the external

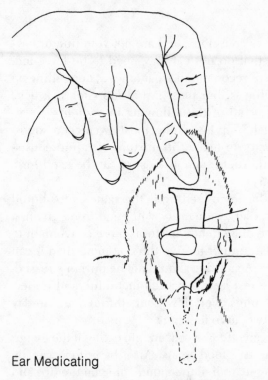

Ear Medicating

ear canal with the right hand, expel the medication, and then gently massage the outside of the ear canal to distribute the medication throughout the ear canal. Dogs usually shake their heads vigorously after medication is put into their ears, so do this treatment outdoors if possible.

The veterinarian may recommend cleaning out the ear canal daily or every few days before inserting the medication (*see* Chapter 6, The Ears; Ear Cleaning and Hair Removal).

Eye Medicating

Ointments are used more commonly than liquids for eye medications in treating dogs because they are easier to apply and are longer lasting. To put medication in a dog's eye, steady the dog's head by placing the left hand under the muz-

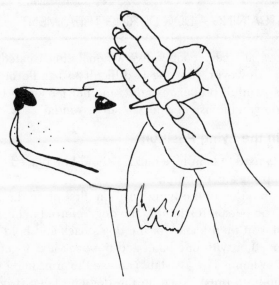

Eye Medicating

zle and place the left thumb at the base of the lower eyelid of the eye to be treated. It is helpful if a second person can hold the dog. Roll the lower eyelid down with the left thumb to create a cul-de-sac between the inside of the eyelid (conjunctiva) and the eyeball. With the right hand resting on the side of the dog's face behind the eye to be treated, and the medication being held between the thumb and index finger, place the medication into the cul-de-sac. Close the eyelid quickly and gently massage it to distribute the medication over the eye surface. Try not to allow the tip of the medication container to touch the eye because this could injure the eye, or become contaminated and spread an infection (if present) to the other eye.

RESTRAINING A DOG DURING TREATMENT

Most dogs are very cooperative when being treated by their owner. However, if a dog is difficult to handle or the treatment is painful, proper restraint, another person to hold the dog, and even the use of a muzzle are essential.

Restraint in the Lying Position

If a dog is hard to handle, a muzzle should be placed on it before attempting any restraint.

To restrain a dog in the lying position, first place the dog on its side. The person restraining the dog, referred to here as the assistant, can then lean over the dog's back and hold the front legs together with one hand and the back legs together with the other hand. The assistant can use the arms and even the upper body to press down on the dog and keep it lying flat.

It is always helpful to place dogs on a table for treatments because they feel less secure at this height, and as a result they struggle less. It is easy to lift a small dog by placing one

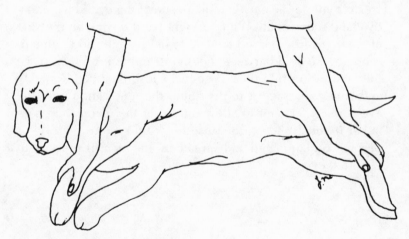

Restraint in the Lying Position

hand under the chest and the other under the hind legs or under the abdomen. To lift a large dog place one arm under the abdomen and the other under the chest or around the front of the chest. Working at table height is also a great deal easier on the assistant's back. Additionally, the person doing the treatment can do a much better job when working at table height. Kind words, petting, coaxing, gentleness, and before-and-after-treatment food treats, all help to make the job easier.

An even safer technique, if the dog has not been muzzled and there is a chance it will bite during the treatment, is to have the assistant use one hand to hold the mouth of the dog closed, and the other hand to hold the front legs together. The assistant can then use the arm holding the front legs and the upper body to press the dog down and keep it lying flat.

Restraint in the Sitting Position

To restrain a dog in the sitting position, stand it, preferably on a table, and have the assistant place one arm under the dog's throat and around the neck. The other arm should be placed over the dog's back and around the abdomen. Pressure can then be applied to the dog's rear back area with the assistant's shoulder, which will force and hold the dog in a sitting position.

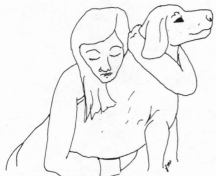

Restraint in the Sitting Position

Restraint in the Standing Position

To restrain a dog in the standing position, the assistant should place one arm under the dog's throat and around the neck. The other arm is then placed under the dog's abdomen and over the back. Slight upward pressure is applied to the lower abdomen to keep the dog in a standing position.

Muzzling a Dog

Muzzling a dog is not unkind, and considering some dogs have three hundred pounds of biting pressure in their jaws, it is a good precaution before attempting painful or unpleasant treatments. Even the best-tempered of dogs may bite its owner, not deliberately, but as a reflex, if it is being hurt. Most dogs do not have trouble breathing when muzzled, although a tight muzzle should not be left on for long periods as it can cause discomfort and lead to respiratory problems.

Muzzles can be purchased at pet stores, but unless the dog owner is doing a lot of treatments, a homemade muzzle is just

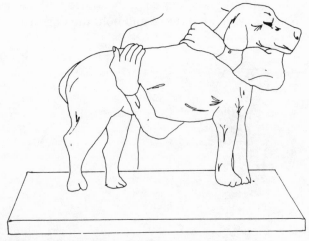

Restraint in the Standing Position

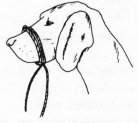 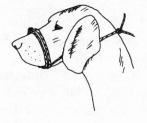

Technique for Muzzling

as satisfactory and not difficult to make. A muzzle can be made using a bandage or a soft rope. Tie the bandage around the muzzle (nose and chin) by placing it under the chin and looping it over the nose. Then bring it under the chin and loop again. Pull the ends behind the ears and double-knot them. The muzzle should be tight enough so that the dog cannot open its mouth, but not so tight that it is cutting into the skin and hurting the dog. It is more difficult to muzzle pug-nosed dogs because they have pushed-in faces, but it can be done, although with these breeds it is important not to leave the muzzles on for too long as these dogs do tend to have trouble breathing when muzzled.

HOME TREATMENTS

Home treatments for medical problems in dogs have been described throughout this book and are listed by page number in the index at the back of the book. Included here is additional information on first-aid treatment for some of the more frequently encountered medical problems in dogs.

Minor Wounds

Provided they are not extensive, and do not need stitches and are not deep punctures which may result in serious infections, wounds can be readily treated by the dog owner. They should be washed well with mild soap and water, and any embedded dirt or debris should be flushed out. Following this, a skin antiseptic such as 3% hydrogen peroxide or Betadine should be applied to the wound.

If the wound is infected and draining pus, it needs to be kept open and flushed out daily until there is no further drainage. Additionally, over-the-counter antibiotic ointment can be inserted into and around the wound twice daily to control the infection.

Any wound that does not start to heal in a few days should be attended to by a veterinarian, as there may be a foreign body (such as a grass awn) in the wound or the deeper tissues may be infected. Wounds that penetrate the full thickness of the skin and are over one inch long should be sutured by your veterinarian as soon after the injury as possible to prevent scarring and infection.

Bandaging

Bandaging is not recommended because dogs tend to tear bandages off, and wounds heal faster if exposed to the air. Wounds that are exposed to contamination, such as foot wounds, and those that the dog constantly licks or scratches, will need to be bandaged.

Following treatment of the wound, a sterile gauze pad should be placed over it; it can then be wrapped in a bandage. Because dogs tend to remove bandages, further reinforcement with adhesive tape is advisable and also helps to keep the bandage dry. Bandages, particularly on the limbs, must not be applied too tightly or they may cut off blood circulation, which can lead to gangrene. Bandages should be removed every few days in order to check the wound and re-treat it.

Elizabethan Collar

As the name implies, these are large, flat, wide restraint collars designed to prevent dogs from tearing with their teeth at wounds on the body and the feet, or using their nails to

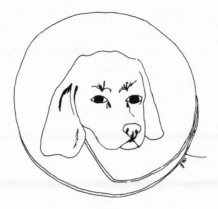

Elizabethan Collar

scratch their head, eyes, and ears. They are available from veterinarians and some pet stores, and come in sizes to fit all dogs. Many dog owners make these collars out of cardboard, because the commercial collars are usually made of plastic and are fairly expensive.

Bleeding

A pressure pad, such as gauze pads, a clean cloth, or even paper towels, should be used to control any external bleeding in a dog. Press the pad gently over the bleeding wound for a few minutes until the bleeding stops. If the bleeding does not stop, bandage over the pressure pad if the wound is in an area which can be bandaged. If this does not control the bleeding, keep applying a pressure pad and seek veterinary emergency care. If bleeding is controlled, leave the wound alone, or leave the bandage on for twelve hours and then treat it as a minor wound. However, if the wound starts bleeding again at this point, it is best to have a veterinarian tend to it.

Tourniquet

Severe bleeding of a limb or the tail can be controlled with a tourniquet if the pressure pad technique is not effective. Apply the tourniquet, which can be rope, string, bandage, or

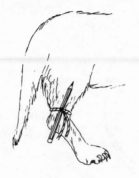

Method of Applying a Tourniquet

whatever is available, about 3 or 4 inches above the bleeding wound, as tightly as necessary to stop the bleeding. It helps to put a stick or pencil through the knot loop and use this to twist and tighten the tourniquet until bleeding is controlled. Any wound bleeding enough to require a tourniquet should receive emergency veterinary treatment. The tourniquet should be opened for one minute every 15 minutes to allow the limb tissues to be oxygenated. Tourniquets are to be avoided if possible because they frequently lead to later complications and even to loss of a limb if they are left on too long or put on too tightly.

Postsurgical Wounds and Sutures (Stitches)

Dogs sent home from the veterinary hospital with stitches in a wound should be checked daily to be sure that the wound is healing and not infected. If there is any swelling, redness, or a watery or pustular discharge, the dog should be returned to the hospital. If a dog continually licks the wound or tries to bite through the stitches, report this to the veterinarian, as it may be necessary to tranquilize the dog, bandage the wound, or use a restraint collar. Skin stitches need to be removed in ten days to two weeks, at which time the dog should be returned to the hospital unless the dog owner has arranged to remove the stitches at home.

Splints

Most dogs with a broken leg are suffering from shock or other serious injuries, so it is best to seek immediate emergency veterinary care rather than spend time putting on a splint. A broken limb can be supported with a pillow or even a towel while transporting the dog to the veterinary hospital; if the dog is in severe pain, it may be necessary to muzzle it for safety.

If veterinary care is not immediately available, a splint can be applied to a broken limb after the dog has been restrained and also preferably muzzled. Bleeding must be controlled first, and any open wound should be covered with sterile gauze pads. Straighten the limb as much as possible without causing the dog too much pain. Use cardboard or newspapers to wrap and support the leg, or use a flat stick on each side of the leg, and overwrap whichever of these splint materials are used with bandages or tape to immobilize the limb. Do not wrap so tightly that circulation is cut off.

Dehydration

Dehydration is the condition that results from excessive loss of body water. It leads to serious medical problems and usually accompanies severe illnesses, fever, vomiting, and diarrhea. A dehydrated dog will have dry gums and eyes, and the eyes will appear sunken. To further identify dehydration

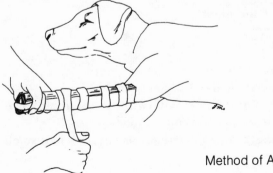

Method of Applying a Splint

in a dog, lift the skin up over the upper back, and if it does not spring back to its normal position at once, this indicates the dog is dehydrated. The longer it takes for the skin to return to its normal position, the more dehydrated the dog is. Most dehydrated dogs will need to be given intravenous or subcutaneous fluids by the veterinarian, but force-feeding water will help to lessen the dehydration until you can reach a veterinary hospital. A vomiting dog should not, of course, be force-fed water.

WHEN IT IS NECESSARY TO SEE A VETERINARIAN

Dogs, like people, have good days and bad days with regard to how they feel, so minor changes in mood or appetite are not significant, nor is an occasional bout of vomiting or diarrhea. However, if any of the following signs of illness occur, it is time to take the dog to the veterinarian:

SYMPTOMS OF MINOR ILLNESS OR EARLY SYMPTOMS OF SERIOUS ILLNESS

- Appetite—loss of appetite for more than one day or change in appetite.
- Behavior—quieter than usual for a few days.
- Drinking—excessive (This is normal if the surrounding temperature is high.)
- Urination—excessive.
- Fever—104° Fahrenheit.

SYMPTOMS OF SERIOUS ILLNESS

- Appetite—complete loss of appetite.
- Weight Loss—gradual or sudden weight loss.
- Vomiting—vomiting more than twice, or continuing over more than one day, or if vomit is bloody.
- Diarrhea—diarrhea for more than one day, or if foul-smelling or bloody.

- Urination—excessive urination, none, or straining to urinate.
- Dehydration—recognizable by sunken and dry eyes, a dry mouth, and loss of elasticity of the skin (if pulled up over back, does not spring back at once).
- Fever—over 104° Fahrenheit.
- Behavior—severe depression or hyperexcitability.
- Pain—signs of pain are usually obvious in dogs.
- Gums—white or bluish appearance to gums.
- Heart Rate—heart rate increased or decreased from normal, or weak or irregular.
- Respiratory Rate—breathing rate increased or decreased from normal, or labored breathing.
- Muscle Tremors—shivering or muscle quivers.
- Convulsion (Seizures)—also called fits.
- Paralysis—cannot move body or one or more limbs.

EMERGENCIES

- Cardiac or Respiratory Arrest.
- All Serious Accidents and Injuries.
- Unconsciousness.
- Shock.
- Poisonings or Suspected Poisonings.
- Hemorrhaging—uncontrollable bleeding, external or internal.
- Fractures.
- Eclampsia (Milk Fever).
- Anaphylaxis—severe allergic reaction.
- Stomach Torsion and Dilation.
- Continuous Seizures (Convulsions).

19

You and Your Veterinarian

Good communications are essential in the relationship between veterinarian and dog owner. An understanding on the dog owner's part of what is involved in becoming a veterinarian and what small-animal veterinary practice is all about is a good first step in developing an open, trusting, and gratifying relationship with a veterinarian. The following brief overview is included to introduce the dog owner to these subjects, and some helpful suggestions are also included on choosing a veterinarian and on being a good veterinary client.

VETERINARY MEDICINE

Doctor of Veterinary Medicine Degree

Doctors of veterinary medicine or DVMs (some are VMDs), called veterinarians, receive university training equivalent to that of human medical doctors, or MDs. Two years of undergraduate studies are required to enter veterinary school, but most students entering veterinary school today have bachelor's degrees in science, and many have a master's or a PhD. Until recently, the public seemed to assume that veterinarians were second-class doctors, and that the study of veterinary medicine was not nearly as difficult as that of human medicine. Probably this myth grew up because the value of animal life is considered to be less important than that of human life. In reality, there is no difference between human or animal medical studies; medicine is medicine, and in some ways the veterinary courses are more difficult because so many different animals have to be covered.

Once students receive their DVM degree, they must then pass state board examinations for each state they wish to practice in. Internships or residencies are not required of veterinarians, although now many do join research veterinary hospitals on graduation for one or more years of additional studies and clinical experience. Most other new graduate veterinarians who intend to become practitioners join the staff of a veterinary hospital as salaried employees, to gain clinical and business experience prior to opening their own practices.

Number of Veterinarians

There are twenty-nine fully accredited veterinary schools in the United States and Canada. The acceptance rate for applicants is about one out of ten, versus one out of six for human medical schools. There are 37,500 DVMs and 450,000 MDs in the U.S. By the year 2000, it is projected there will be over 60,000 veterinarians. About 15% of veterinarians are women, but close to 50% of veterinary students are now women. In twenty-five years or so, the male/female distribution is expected to be 50/50.

Veterinary Careers

Veterinarians are trained mainly to look after the health and welfare of domestic animals and pets. The veterinarian most familiar to the city dweller is the small-animal practitioner who runs a pet hospital, either alone or with one or more colleagues. Less well known veterinary careers, of perhaps greater social significance, exist in the fields of disease prevention, meat inspection, and medical research.

About 75% of veterinarians are in practice, treating domestic animals and pets. Some practitioners treat only one species

of animal, for example, equine-only or feline-only practitioners. The remaining 25% of veterinarians work in poultry medicine, teaching, research, laboratory animal medicine, wildlife
medicine, zoo animal medicine, fur-bearing animal medicine,
aquatic medicine, avian (bird) medicine, industry (drug and
equipment manufacture), public health, and in the military
forces.

Many veterinarians are now specializing, similarly to
human medical doctors, and are continuing their studies for a
number of years after graduation. They are studying to become board-certified veterinary ophthalmologists, dermatolo-
gists, cardiologists, neurologists, oncologists, etc.

Veterinary Practice

Modern veterinary hospitals and clinics offer services and
facilities directly comparable to human hospitals. No veterinary hospital can afford a million-dollar computerized x-ray
machine or laser beam equipment, but all the basic medical,
surgical, anesthetic, and laboratory equipment found in a
human hospital is available in the average up-to-date veterinary hospital.

The staff of a veterinary hospital will include one or more
veterinarians, animal health technicians (equivalent to nurses
in human medicine), on-the-job-trained veterinary assistants,
animal caretakers, and office and management personnel. Veterinary hospitals are designed to include waiting room(s), examination rooms, an x-ray room, a laboratory, a pharmacy, a
library, one or more offices, surgeries, treatment rooms, kennels, exercise runs, intensive care units, supply rooms, a
kitchen, isolation quarters for contagious diseases, and many
have an apartment for a twenty-four-hour caretaker.

The costs of setting up in practice are much higher for
veterinarians than MDs, because veterinarians require their
own hospitals and do not have a centralized local hospital to
which to send their patients. Each veterinary practitioner
needs to be business-oriented as well, and as any human hos-

pital administrator will tell you, running a hospital is not an easy job. Thus, in some ways a veterinary career is more complicated than a career in human medicine, and certainly it is much more difficult to start a practice because of the high initial investment needed to acquire property, and to build and equip a hospital.

Veterinary practitioners spend about 50% of their time in consultation with clients during office calls. These consultations include discussions on general health care of the pet and its diet, preventive vaccination administration, explaining illnesses, and treatments of minor illnesses and injuries. The other 50% of the time is spent treating hospitalized patients, doing diagnostic tests, and performing surgeries, which can include anything from elective surgeries such as spays and castrations, to tumor removal, fracture repair, or removing an intestinal obstruction. If emergencies arise, they will take precedence over the more routine daily schedule. For this reason, veterinary waiting rooms sometimes become overcrowded and appointments are not kept on time.

Veterinarians are expected to offer twenty-four-hour emergency service to their clients, and this is one reason there is a trend toward larger group practices. No veterinarian in practice alone can be available twenty-four hours a day, 365 days a year, although many do work sixty hours and more a week, and additionally cover emergency night and weekend calls. A recent trend in many medium- to-large-sized cities is the emergency veterinary clinic. These clinics are open to handle emergencies outside of regular hospital hours. Not all veterinary hospitals refer emergency cases to these clinics; some continue to offer their own emergency service. When the pet owner uses one of these emergency clinics, the pet will receive immediate emergency treatment, but will be transferred back to the owner's veterinarian for continuing care. These emergency clinics are appreciated by the pet-owning public when a genuine emergency arises in the middle of the night. Another advantage is that the pet owner does not have to call and disturb his or her own veterinarian, which can be, and often is, embarrassing if there is no real emergency or the problem turns out to be a minor one.

Animal Health Technicians

Animal Health Technicians (AHTs) are the veterinary equivalent of the human health services' nurses. For anyone who likes working with animals, but does not have the ambition or inclination to become a veterinarian, this is an excellent alternative career choice. The AHT program was developed in 1970, and involves a two-year, college-level course of training, together with practical experience gained by working in a veterinary hospital.

AHTs are trained in the care and handling of animals, and they work under the supervision of a veterinarian. Their duties include nursing care of animals, recording case information, preparing animals and instruments for surgery, assisting in surgery, laboratory work, medicating, dressing wounds, medical procedures, taking x-rays, ordering and stocking supplies, and communicating with veterinary clients about their pets' care, handling, vaccination schedules, and illnesses.

Not all veterinary hospitals have trained AHTs, as this is a relatively new field. On-the-job-trained veterinary assistants also work with and care for animals in the veterinary hospital.

CHOOSING A VETERINARIAN

The average dog owner today is well informed and interested in his or her dog's health and medical care and wants to know how to keep it healthy, what to feed it, what is the diagnosis if it is ill, how this diagnosis is made, how the illness will be treated, what the prognosis is, and what the cost of treatment will be. Thus, good communication is the most important quality a dog owner looks for when choosing a veterinarian.

A survey of veterinary practitioners showed that their success in practice depended on the following, in descending order of importance: an ability to communicate well with their clients; the hospital's appearance and cleanliness; the hospital's location; the appearance and behavior of the staff; the staff's attitude to animals; the fees; and the availability of emergency services.

If you acquire a dog or move to a new area with your dog, it is important to arrange for veterinary care at once. It is difficult to locate and choose a veterinarian under emergency circumstances, and many veterinarians will not accept emergency calls unless the dog owner is an established client.

In choosing a veterinarian, the following points are of importance:

1. It is essential that the pet owner likes dealing with the veterinarian and that communications between them go well. If either of these qualities is missing, another veterinarian should be sought.

2. The best way to find a good veterinarian is to have one recommended by a conscientious pet owner.

3. Make an evaluation of the hospital's appearance, the staff, and the service. If interested, pet owners can ask for a prearranged tour of the hospital, because no well-run hospital will refuse.

4. Discuss fees openly. If the veterinarian will not discuss fees, work within a budget, or gives the pet owner large bills without explaining the services rendered, it is time to find another veterinarian. It is also advisable to find out the credit policy of the hospital before incurring charges you cannot pay. Many veterinary hospitals have a cash- and credit card-only policy, and will no longer open charge accounts. Unfortunately, too many bad debts brought about these policies.

5. Talk to the others in the waiting room. This is an excellent way to get a feeling for the type of clientele the hospital is attracting. Are they concerned and responsible pet owners, and are they happy with the service they are receiving?

6. Ask about emergency service. Is it available or is an emergency clinic recommended?

7. A hospital should keep pet owners fully informed on their dogs' progress while hospitalized. Usually the owner is asked to check in at a specific time each day, as it is difficult for the hospital to contact each owner on a daily basis.

8. Telephone calls to the veterinarian should be answered or returned promptly, or at a specified time if the veterinarian is in consultation or performing surgery.

9. A dog should be sent home from the hospital in a clean condition, and with full, preferably written, instructions on continuing home care.

10. The staff should be courteous and friendly. For instance, do they call dogs by their names?

11. Appointments should be kept on time. If an emergency has backed up appointments, an apology should be offered along with a brief explanation.

12. A veterinarian should be fully cooperative in getting a second opinion if one is asked for.

13. A veterinarian should also be willing to refer a dog to another veterinarian if the case demands specialized work outside his or her area of training.

BEING A GOOD VETERINARY CLIENT

As important as choosing the right veterinarian is learning to be a good veterinary client. In reality the two go together. Basically, good communications and good manners are all that are needed to make the veterinarian/client relationship satisfactory. The ideal veterinary client will:

1. Keep good records on his or her dog's medical history.

2. Make appointments and arrive for them on time.

3. Use the office call to discuss the dog's care or illness, not as a social occasion.

4. Ask questions if there is difficulty understanding any aspect of the dog's illness or medical care.

5. Pay bills on time.

6. Discuss fees openly, and let the veterinarian know if the treatment suggested is not affordable. Alternative treatments that are less expensive can be requested or special arrangements made to pay over a certain period of time.

7. Be sure emergencies are real. Do not call a veterinarian out in the middle of the night for minor ailments or on weekends after the dog has been sick for three days.

8. Be aware that a veterinarian cannot diagnose and treat a dog over the phone, unless it is a question of continuing home care.

9. Follow home care treatments as directed. Be sure to call or return the dog to the hospital if the condition worsens or there is a problem with administration of the medication.

10. See a veterinarian yearly for booster vaccinations for the dog, a physical examination, and routine teeth care.

11. Bring the dog in early if signs of illness occur, but make an appointment first unless it is a genuine emergency such as an accident or poisoning.

12. Discuss problems concerning the dog's illness, the cost of treatments, the method of treatment, etc., with the veterinarian before seeking another opinion. Very often in such instances, it is poor communication or failure to understand the chronic nature of some diseases that causes such problems, and going from one veterinarian to another can be both a waste of time and money. If the problem cannot be resolved, ask for a second opinion before changing veterinarians, as this is less costly and straightens out most difficulties.

Appendix A

ACUPUNCTURE

Acupuncture means "piercing of points" and is claimed to be successful in all species for treating certain medical problems. The most common application in the western world has been for the relief of pain. There is now a National Association for Veterinary Acupuncture.

Technique

Acupuncture can be defined as the stimulation of specific points, or areas, of the surface of humans or animals to obtain treatment, pain relief, or anesthetic effects. Only certain areas of the surface of an animal are susceptible to acupuncture effects. Experienced acupuncturists can recognize these points by touch, but most users of the technique in the United States rely on anatomical charts to locate them.

Today, stainless steel needles are used to stimulate specific points in various locations, depending on what treatment or effect needs to be achieved. Most animals accept treatment fairly readily. Other methods of stimulation presently used include infrared radiation, drug injections, electrostimulation, massage, and the use of magnetic fields.

Application in Dogs

Treatment usually takes from twenty to forty minutes per session. Sessions may be as frequent as two to three times a day, or as seldom as once a week; often these are done over long periods of time, depending on the condition being treated. In dogs, success has been achieved using acupuncture in many diseases and conditions, including epilepsy; whiplash injuries; paralysis; lameness; shock; arthritic conditions; and abnormal behaviors, such as aggression.

Acupuncture Does Not Cure Disease

It must be remembered that while acupuncture can often relieve disease symptoms, it cannot correct the basic cause of the disease. Other standard medical or surgical methods must be used to treat or cure the disease or condition; if this is not possible, and the disease is chronic or progressive, acupuncture may help to relieve the symptoms, particularly the pain, and improve the quality of life for the dog.

ANESTHESIA

Anesthesia is a state of unconsciousness brought about by the use of anesthetic agents that produce controlled reversible depression of the nervous system. These agents are given by intravenous injection (directly into the bloodstream), inhalation of a gas, or rarely, by other injection routes or by mouth. Anesthesia is used in veterinary medicine to control pain and relax muscles during surgery, restrain animals during treatment or other medical procedures, and treat convulsions; and for euthanasia.

Dogs are anesthetized more often than people because it is difficult to restrain them during such medical procedures as suturing a wound, taking an x-ray, or cleaning the teeth. Anesthesia is also a more humane approach to treating dogs because they cannot, of course, understand why they are being restrained and treated; even if the pain has been controlled with drugs, they still interpret the experience as unnecessary punishment.

When an anesthetic is given, there is loss of consciousness, the muscles relax, the heart and respiratory rate slow down, the temperature drops, and all body systems are depressed. In this state the body is only one level above death, and this is why anesthesia carries with it some risk. Unfortunately, anesthetic dosage is not an exact science and the response of different dogs of the same weight to the same dosage is often different. This is why anesthesiology is considered an art as well as a science. The risk of overdosage or unforeseen reactions to an anesthetic is not high in veterinary medicine because veterinarians are highly trained in anesthesiology: they use anesthetics daily; they closely monitor the respiratory rate, heart rate, blood pressure, and reflexes during anesthesia; and they constantly adjust the dosage to keep the animal pain-free and relaxed but not too deeply anesthetized.

However, despite the best equipment, assistants, techniques, highly trained and experienced veterinarians, and a careful pre-anesthetic examination of all patients, an occasional anesthetic death will occur in every veterinary hospital. Most deaths are in high-risk patients—animals that are seriously ill, weak, injured, obese, very old, or suffering from respiratory or heart disease—that require anesthesia. Surgery itself, except for some very complicated surgeries, is seldom the cause of an animal's death. The major risks are from the anesthetic or the development of shock.

Dog owners readily understand if a sick dog dies when undergoing major surgery, but few understand if an apparently healthy dog dies while having its teeth cleaned or is being spayed. Seldom is such a death the fault of the veterinarian or the veterinary hospital. Despite medical advances and a low mortality rate, anesthesia still carries with it risks that cannot be avoided. One out of approximately every 10,000 dogs undergoing anesthesia will die of anesthetic-related causes. Considering the number of animals that are anesthetized daily in veterinary hospitals throughout the country, this is an excellent record, and the veterinary profession should be admired for its competence in this area of medicine. Dog owners need not be overly concerned when their pets need anesthesia but should be aware that there is some risk. Fortunately, as in so many other medical treatments, the benefits definitely outweigh the risks. Anesthesia is one of the most humane aspects of veterinary medicine; people are not so lucky, they have to go through many unpleasant medical procedures while fully conscious!

EUTHANASIA

Euthanasia, also referred to by pet owners as "putting the animal to sleep," is defined as an easy or painless death, or as mercy killing, which is the deliberate ending of life of a person or animal suffering from an incurable and painful disease. As the life span of dogs and cats is so much shorter than that of humans, most pet owners will be faced with the decision, at some time, of whether or not to euthanize a pet.

The pet owner always makes the decision on whether or not to euthanize the pet, but the veterinarian advises. The primary consideration should be what is best for the pet. Ideally, euthanasia is suggested if an old or diseased pet has ceased to enjoy life and the possibilities of it ever enjoying life again, even with medical intervention, are remote. The pet owner is more aware of the enjoyment-of-life criteria, and the veterinarian of the prognosis, so it is really a joint decision.

Unfortunately, there are many abuses of euthanasia, and pet lovers would be horrified if they were aware of some of the reasons veterinary clients give for requesting euthanasia for a pet. Most veterinarians refuse to euthanize a healthy animal unless it is vicious or dangerous. However, the humane societies and city pounds have become dumping grounds for irresponsible pet owners, and these organizations are forced to destroy many healthy animals daily. Recent figures from the U.S. Department of Agriculture estimate twenty million dogs and cats a year are no longer wanted.

Veterinary euthanasia is done with the administration of an anesthetic, either by injection or with the use of a gas (inhalation) anesthetic. Once the animal is sedated, an overdose is given to ensure that it will not recover consciousness again. This technique of euthanasia is entirely painless, except for the prick of the needle if an injection is used, as anyone who has ever had an anesthetic for surgery can attest. Many pet owners are concerned that their pets will not be euthanized, as requested, but will be used for research or experiments. If a pet owner requests euthanasia and the veterinarian agrees to do it, then by law the veterinarian must perform this service. Pet owners can stay with their pet while it is being euthanized, or if they do not care for this, they can ask to see the remains after the pet is dead, to relieve any anxieties they may have. Furthermore, if a pet is to be used for research, the pet owner must request this and give permission in writing. The veterinarian may suggest this course, for example, if an owner can no longer afford or does not want to go on with medical care, while the veterinarian does not want to give up on the pet. The veterinarian then requests permission to continue treatment at no charge or to use some experimental treatments on the animal. The owner's permission must be given in writing.

After euthanasia veterinarians usually dispose of the remains by cremation, although the method depends to some degree on state law. A number of remains are cremated at one time, so it is not possible to give the individual ashes to the pet owner. The remains are not used for research, unless this is specifically requested by the owner, or asked for in writing by the veterinarian. Most states no longer allow pet owners to bury the bodies themselves, but many states now have cremation services for pets through private enterprises or the humane societies, and the pet owner is given the ashes in an attractive box or urn. Pet cemeteries are also available in most states.

Appendix B

DE-SKUNKING

The time-honored remedy for de-skunking a dog is to flush out the eyes with water and then to wash the dog with soap and water, preferably using a pet detergent shampoo, dry the dog, and then rub tomato juice into the dog's coat and skin. Allow this to dry and then rinse off with plain water. A second application of tomato juice may be necessary.

This is a time-consuming and messy process and many authorities claim that a rinse with a dilute ammonia solution after bathing is just as effective as the tomato juice technique. When the dog dries, the odor will be gone but when the hair is wet, a faint skunk odor may return for weeks after either of these cleanup methods.

There are also a number of commercial products available at pet stores in areas where skunks are prevalent specifically made for de-skunking dogs.

In many western states skunks have been involved in the transmission of rabies, so it is important that the dog's rabies vaccination be up to date. Anyone finding a dead skunk should call the local public health authorities to enquire if they wish to test it for rabies. The skunk should not be handled, particularly with your bare hands.

MOTION SICKNESS

Motion sickness, displayed by salivation, nausea, and vomiting, is not uncommon in dogs and children traveling by car. Although not an emergency situation, it is unpleasant for the dog and inconvenient for the dog owner. Most dogs overcome the sickness as they get accustomed to car travel, but preventive motion sickness medications can be used with success during this adjustment period.

Sedatives, antinausea and antisalivation drugs, and tranquilizers are all effective in controlling the symptoms, and can be obtained from a veterinarian.

Over-the-counter human motion sickness medications, given about thirty minutes before the trip, can be used if an adjustment in dosage is made for the weight of the dog. To avoid the inconvenience of having a dog vomit in the car while waiting for it to outgrow the problem, do not feed the dog for eight hours prior to car travel. Also, daily car trips help a dog to adjust to car travel and will speed up the adjustment period.

TRAVEL AND QUARANTINE

Regulations regarding travel for dogs depend on the mode of transportation and the state or country the dog is being moved to or visiting. Most times the dog will need a recently issued health certificate and a rabies vaccination within the last twelve months. A veterinarian can take care of these items, and will be familiar with the requirements for interstate travel. However, for foreign travel the regulations are constantly changing, so it is best to check with the consulate of the country on the present regulations for importing a dog. The airlines also have regulations which must be met before they will ship a dog, which usually include a health certificate, rabies vaccination certificate, and specifications for the type of cage or container required for shipment.

Some foreign countries and the state of Hawaii have quarantine regulations which vary between three and six months. Dog owners must pay for the dog's boarding during this period.

Index

Thyroid, 82, 254
Ticks, 51–53
Toads, poisonous, 290
Tonsillitis, 247–248
Tourniquet, 265, 331–332
Toxoplasmosis, 45
Trachea, collapse, 164
Tracheitis, 248–251
Tracheobronchitis, 248–251
Tranquilizers, 298
Trauma. *See* specific injury
  brain, 207–209
  nerve, 211–213
  spinal cord, 209–210
  thoracic, 250, 251, 279
Travel, with dog, 350
Treatments. *See* Home Medical
  Care; specific disease
Trichiasis, 95, 164
Tubal ligation, 157
Tuberculosis, 244
Tularemia, 244
Tumors, 259–261
Twitching, 315

Ulcers
  duodenal, 177–178
  eye, 98, 99
  stomach, 177–178
Unconsciousness, 264–269, 315
Uremia, 189
Urinary incontinence, 198, 199

Urinary System Diseases, 187–199
Urination problems, 315
Urolithiasis, 196–198
Urticaria, 64, 65
Uterine diseases, 146–147, 314, 316

Vaccines/Vaccination, 237–243
Vagina, 148
Vasectomy, 159
Veterinarians and Veterinary
  Medicine, 336–343
Veterinary drugs, 295–307
Viral diseases, 238–243, 249–251
Visceral larva migrans, 59
Vision in dogs, 91
Vitamins. *See* Nutrition
Vomiting, 171–173, 294, 309, 316, 349, 350
Vulva, 148

Warts, 169
Weakness, 316
Weaning, 154
Weight loss, 316
Weight reduction. *See* Obesity
Wheezing, 316
Whelping, 151–153
Whipworms, 43–44
Worms, 37–45, 134–139, 299
Wounds, 76, 275–276, 316, 329–330, 332